Essential Skills in Clinical Medicine

Essential Skills in Clinical Medicine

CHARLES L. BARDES, MD
Assistant Professor of Medicine
Cornell University Medical College
Assistant Attending Physician
The New York Hospital—Cornell Medical Center
New York, New York

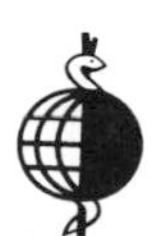

F. A. Davis Company • Philadelphia

F. A. Davis Company
1915 Arch Street
Philadelphia, PA 19103

Printed in the United States of America

Last digit indicates print number: 10 9 8 7 6 5 4 3 2 1

Medical Editor: Robert W. Reinhardt
Medical Developmental Editor: Bernice M. Wissler
Production Editor: Nancee A. Vogel
Cover Designer: Louis J. Forgione

Library of Congress Cataloging in Publication Data

Bardes, Charles L., 1956–
Essential skills in clinical medicine / Charles L. Bardes.
p. cm.
Includes bibliographical references and index.
ISBN 0-8036-0014-3 (pbk.)
1. Clinical medicine—Handbooks, manuals, etc. I. Title.
[DNLM: 1. Clinical Medicine—handbooks. WB 39 B245e 1996]
RC55.B27 1996
616—dc20
DNLM/DLC
for Library of Congress 95-19189
CIP

Has anyone not yet perceived the aim of doctors?
It is this:
that by their care and dedication life and,
moreover, a good life may be sustained.

—Marsilio Ficino, Letters IV.14

Preface

Medical students in the third and fourth years, interns, and residents share a common activity: they perform clinical work. Their work is of two main types: diagnostic problem solving and clinical management. Learners are thrust into this role in the beginning (approximately) of the third year of medical school. They have completed some 2 years of training in basic science, during which they've accumulated an immense number of biomedical facts. But they generally have had almost no guidance as to what clinical life is like—what doctors do and how they think.

This book is a guide to diagnostic reasoning and clinical praxis. Its purpose is to help those learning clinical medicine to become better clinicians. Specifically, the reader should learn:

- How to be an effective clinician; how to do what clinical students, interns, and residents are expected to do.
- How to work up a case: from a problem list, through differential diagnosis and diagnostic testing, to diagnosis. This book does not deal with therapy, which is the subject of numerous instructional manuals.

Part I focuses on practical clinical skills such as navigating the hospital and clinics, writing notes and orders, presenting cases orally, participating in rounds, performing procedures, organizing effectively, and interacting with patients.

Part II concerns ways of assimilating clinical information. Chapter 11 describes how to access the medical literature and emphasizes the importance of reading it critically. Chapter 12 provides an overview for interpreting common diagnostic tests (e.g., blood tests, ECGs, and chest x-rays). Chapter 13 outlines the diagnostic and therapeutic approaches to 15 common clinical problems.

Part III deals with diagnostic problem solving, the process by which the clinician arrives at a diagnosis. Each chapter is devoted to a different step in the diagnostic process: the problem list, differential diagnosis, diagnostic testing, and diagnosis. The final chapter uses 14 clinical cases as a set of hands-on exercises in problem-based learning and clinical problem solving. The reader is asked to go through the cases, to answer questions related to the diagnostic process, and to solve the diagnostic puzzle. Answers to these questions, and discussions of the cases, follow.

This book grew out of experiences in teaching medical students and medical house officers at Cornell University Medical College and The New York Hospital, in New York City. These learners, often armed with an astounding array of biomedical facts, knew all about diseases and treatments but had difficulty applying their knowledge to individual patients. They repeatedly have asked for guidance in making the link between their knowledge and their patients. A course evolved at the medical school, called "Introduction to the Clinical Years," whose purpose has been to provide a bridge between the preclinical and the clinical portions of the medical school curriculum. This book is in large measure an expansion of the themes of that course.

Several of the faculty at Cornell have been instrumental in the development of this volume. Louis J. Aronne, MD, directed the course before me and gave it much of its shape. Joseph G. Hayes, MD, the director of the residency program, has been a paradigm of intelligence, high spirit, and dedication. Intellectual and institutional support have also been provided by Daniel R. Alonso, MD, Mary E. Charlson, MD, and Ralph L. Nachman, MD. At the University of Pennsylvania School of Medicine, where I completed my undergraduate medical studies, Maria Delivoria-Papadopoulos, MD, has stood as a beacon of Hippocratic endeavor and goodness.

To Barbara Lee Kilpatrick, my wife; to John and Emma Bardes, my children; and to Judith Leopold Bardes and Charles Robert Bardes, my parents: all love and gratitude.

Charles L. Bardes, MD

Contents

Part I. The Clinics

Chapter 1. Hospital Organization **3**
The medical team 3
Doctors 3
Other providers 8
The hospital 9

Chapter 2. Ambulatory Settings **11**
Ambulatory medicine: general principles 11
Hospital clinics 14
Neighborhood health centers 16
Physician offices 16
The emergency department 17
The telephone 18

Chapter 3. Rounds **21**
Rounds explained 21
Morning rounds 21
Work rounds 23
Attending rounds 24
"Chart rounds" 25
Sign-out rounds 25
Grand rounds 27
"Roundsmanship" 27

Chapter 4. Writing Notes **29**
General principles 29
Admission notes 35
Progress notes 43
Update notes 44
Procedure notes 44
Surgical notes 47
Discharge notes 49
Outpatient notes 50
Sample admission note 52
Sample progress notes 57

Chapter 5. Oral Presentations **62**
General principles 62
Formal case presentation 63
Presentation on morning rounds 66
Other presentations 69

Chapter 6. Writing Orders **71**
General principles 71
How to write an order 72
Ordering medications 73
Ordering fluids 80
Ordering oxygen 82
Other orders 85
Making sure the order is right 87
Admission orders 88
Daily orders 91
Preoperative orders 92
Postoperative orders 93
Prescriptions 94

Chapter 7. Procedures **99**
Performing procedures 99
Indications and contraindications 100

Complications 101
Informed consent 102
Common procedures 104

Chapter 8. Preventing Nosocomial Infection **107**
General principles 107
Universal precautions 109
Special isolation 111
Preventing injury to oneself 112
Preventing HIV infection 114

Chapter 9. Relations with Patients **117**
Principles 117
Interpersonal relations 118
Ethical responsibilities 122
Legal responsibilities 125

Chapter 10. Being Effective: Goals and Skills **130**
A day in the life 130
On call 131
Being an effective physician-in-training 132

Part II. Assimilating Information

Chapter 11. Accessing the Medical Literature **137**
Sources of information 137
The computer literature search 140
Critical reading 143

Chapter 12. Interpreting Tests **151**
General principles 151

Interpreting blood tests 154
Interpreting chest x-rays 162
Interpreting electrocardiograms 167

Chapter 13. Approaches to Common Clinical Problems **174**
Inpatient problems 175
Outpatient problems 209

Part III. The Diagnostic Process

Chapter 14. The Problem List **231**
Clinical problem solving 231
The problem list: general principles 233
Making the problem list 236

Chapter 15. Differential Diagnosis **240**
General principles 240
Strategies for differential diagnosis 241

Chapter 16. Diagnostic Testing **253**
General principles 253
Test characteristics 255
Using tests 257
Choosing tests 261
Continuous values 263
Combining tests 264
Screening tests 264

Chapter 17. Diagnosis **267**
General principles 267
Diagnosis and decision 272
Problems in diagnosis 274

Chapter 18. Clinical Case Problems 278
Approach to solving clinical cases 278
Case 1: Wilma Trager 281
Case 2: Stetson SanSouci 285
Case 3: Keebler Nobbit 289
Case 4: Dottie Dieffendorfer 295
Case 5: Bartolo Dottore 299
Case 6: Morbia Prendergast 303
Case 7: Eleanor Sniggle 309
Case 8: Omar Deng 317
Case 9: Bunter Frill 323
Case 10: Rex Plover 329
Case 11: Mamie Kriebel 335
Case 12: Hans Castorp 341
Case 13: Ludmilla T. Raum 349
Case 14: Susan Domonas 355

Appendix A. Medical Abbreviations 360

Appendix B. Readings and References 367

Envoi 375

Index 377

PART I

THE CLINICS

CHAPTER 1

Hospital Organization

The Medical Team

1. In the hospital, medical care is delivered by organized units called *medical teams*. The medical team consists of doctors, nurses, nursing assistants or aides, and additional care providers such as social workers, dietitians and physical therapists as well as others. These persons work together to provide the diverse aspects of patient care.

2. Medical students belong to the group of doctors and function as physicians.

Doctors

1. **Intern.** An intern is a physician in the first year of training after medical school. This is called the first post-graduate year, so that an intern is often called a *PGY-1*. The intern has an MD or a DO degree. He or she has usually *not* yet received a medical license and can't practice independently. Interns are authorized to practice medicine under the auspices of the hospital that employs them.

   Interns are the primary link between the patient and the doctors. All patients involved with the house staff have an intern, usually the intern who admitted them initially.

The group of patients assigned to an intern may range in number from 5 to 20 or more, depending on the type of service.

An intern's primary responsibilities include:

Patient Care

- Admitting the patient and performing a complete history and physical examination
- Interviewing and examining each patient at least once daily, and more often if needed
- Interpreting all medical data for each patient
- Making a plan for diagnosis, treatment, discharge, and follow-up
- Coordinating the input from all caregivers

Documentation

- Writing up the admission history and physical examination.
- Writing daily progress notes.
- Writing orders. In most hospitals, the intern writes virtually all the orders for his or her patients.

Nuts and Bolts

- **Procedures.** These may include venipuncture, intravenous catheter insertion, special tests, diagnostic or therapeutic maneuvers, transport, or anything else that a patient requires. While support staff may be assigned to perform some of these functions, it is the intern's responsibility to see that they are done, and done properly.
- **Administration.** This may include ordering tests, calling for results, completing forms, writing prescriptions, etc.

2. **Resident.** A resident is a physician who has com-

pleted an internship and is engaged in training for a specialty, such as internal medicine or ophthalmology. A resident usually obtains a medical license during the PGY-2 year. Residents are responsible for supervising interns' and students' clinical work as well as for teaching.

A resident's duties include:

- Making rounds daily with interns and students.
- Overseeing patient care. The resident follows all patients belonging to the interns and students under his or her supervision.
- Creating an academic environment. The resident has an opportunity to read and analyze the current literature pertaining to the clinical problems at hand. The resident is responsible for sharing his or her findings in a meaningful way with the interns and students, who have less opportunity for inquiry.

Together, interns and residents are called *house officers* and comprise the *graduate staff* of the hospital. The term *residency* is sometimes applied to both the PGY-1 and subsequent years, and sometimes to the postinternship years only. Used in the former sense, residencies range from 3 years, for fields such as internal medicine, to 8 years, for fields such as neurosurgery.

3. **Fellow.** A fellow has completed residency and is engaged in subspecialty training. For example, a renal fellow has completed a residency in internal medicine and is now training as a nephrologist. Subspecialty medical teams may include fellows; for example, the Coronary Intensive Care Unit is likely to have a cardiology fellow. Otherwise, fellows are more likely to function as consultants.
4. **Attending.** An attending is a physician who has completed training. The attending physician supervises and coordinates all aspects of care, and also bears the ultimate responsibility for the patient. In

teaching hospitals, the attendings are often faculty members of the medical college. Attendings may also be community physicians who admit to the hospital.

All patients have an attending physician. If the patient has a preexisting relation with a personal physician, that physician becomes the attending during hospitalization. If the patient doesn't have a preexisting relation with a personal physician, the patient is assigned an attending on admission. Physicians admitting to the hospital generally take turns in assuming the responsibility for new patients. In teaching hospitals, the assigned physician is usually the attending who is teaching on a given service at that time. Such a physician is called the *teaching attending*, or the *service attending*.

In the old days, before the 1960s, patients who did not have personal physicians were often admitted under the care of residents and students. An attending, if connected to the case at all, usually supervised from a distance or contributed educational points. The unspoken agreement was that patients received care that was free or inexpensive—but provided by physicians-in-training. These patients were often poor and did not have access to well-qualified personal physicians.

Since the 1960s, the principle has gradually developed that every patient should receive high-quality medical care, at least during hospitalization. The idea that the poor should be subject to unsupervised care by trainees is unacceptable, and illegal. Now, every patient has an attending.

Two vestiges of the old system persist to a variable degree according to institution and individual personalities. Older hospital buildings may have been constructed with separate areas for "private" and "service" patients; the private areas were generally more comfortable and spacious. Newer hospitals usually do not have separate areas. If you work in an older building, the bricks and mortar may retain the fossilized remains of the old system, with four-bedded rooms in some places and two-bedded rooms in others.

More significantly, the relation between the physicians and the patient is slightly different when the attending physician has a personal relation with the patient, compared with when the attending does not. *In all instances, the student, intern, and resident are expected to evaluate patients under their care and to make decisions about management.* This is true whether the patient has a personal attending or a service attending. However, the student and intern sometimes take somewhat more initiative when the attending is a service attending. The service attending, that is, often takes the role of copilot, rather than pilot.

There may be several attending physicians who share in the care of the patient. For example, a patient with heart disease who undergoes surgery may be seen by a cardiologist and the surgeon. One attending, however, is the *attending of record*, the physician who bears ultimate responsibility for the patient's care.

5. **Consultant.** A consultant is a physician who advises the primary team regarding specialty or subspecialty care. The cardiologist who visits the surgical patient is functioning as a consultant. A physician at any level of training, from student to attending, can function as a consultant. The consultant usually doesn't write orders or make the final decisions, but rather makes recommendations.
6. **Medical Students.** Students adopt the roles of interns, to a greater or lesser degree. Early in the third-year *clerkships*, students are not expected to assume the full responsibilities of an intern, and the patient has an intern as well. Late in the clerkships,

the intern tends to fade from view. In the *subinternship* or *practicing internship*, which usually takes place in the fourth year, the student functions as a full-fledged intern, albeit with a lighter patient load than full interns. Patients assigned to a subintern will not also have an intern.

7. The team may include *physician extenders*, professionals who do not have the MD or DO degree but who are trained in the assessment and management of patients. *Physician assistants* and *surgical assistants* have completed a 2- or 3-year program after the bachelor degree and function as interns under specifically outlined circumstances. *Nurse practitioners* and *nurse clinicians* have completed a 1- to 3-year program after the nursing degree and function similarly to physician assistants.
8. There is a balance of responsibility among the doctors on the team. At each level of training, the more capably one performs, the more independence and responsibility one is granted. By taking the initiative with your patients, providing them with excellent care, and participating in the work of the team, you indicate your readiness to interpret medical information and to make decisions.

Other Providers

1. *Nurses* have the responsibility of providing direct patient care, including evaluating patients, participating in planning, and administering treatment. Nurses are highly trained and are not simply technical followers of physician orders. They spend more time with the patient and the family than most physicians, and they see the patient from a special perspective. Their understanding of a patient's situation can provide a crucial contribution to care, and they should be welcomed into the decision-making process. In addition, experienced

nurses often know more about management and therapy than do physicians-in-training, so that they can help you when you're unsure what to do.

2. *Nursing assistants* or *aides* provide relatively unskilled types of care. They may take vital signs, provide personal assistance, help the patient in bathing and toileting, and generally help out. They too spend more time with some patients than you will and may be able to tell you about the patient's needs, level of functioning, state of mind, and social situation.
3. *Social workers* perform two types of service. On the one hand, they offer psychological support and often psychotherapy. On the other, they are the administrative links to services such as entitlement programs, medical assistance, home care, discharge planning, and to patient transfer to rehabilitation centers, nursing homes, or other care facilities.
4. A variety of other providers may be part of the health-care team. *Dietitians* interpret patients' nutritional needs, recommend dietary modifications, and discuss diet with patients. *Physical therapists* and *occupational therapists* assist patients in overcoming musculoskeletal and neurologic deficits. *Phlebotomists* are technicians who draw blood samples. A variety of *technicians* or nurses may also perform electrocardiograms, insert intravenous catheters, educate patients with special needs, etc.
5. A number of administrative personnel, including clerks, messengers, and various levels of managers and supervisors, are also part of the medical team.

The Hospital

1. The teams described above are grouped together according to medical specialty. These groupings of teams are called *services*: the medical service, the surgical service, the psychiatry service, and so on.

Typically, each specialty and subspecialty has its own service.

2. Each team generally assumes responsibility for 10 to 50 patients. The teams may be organized according to subspecialty, geographic location within the hospital, or groupings of attending physicians.

   Example

   Hospital A has a large number of surgical patients. These are divided into the cardiothoracic team, the ophthalmology team, the otorhinolaryngology team, and three general surgery teams.

   Example

   Hospital B has three floors in the S building for pediatric patients, called S-4, S-5, and S-6. Each floor has its own team.

   Example

   Hospital C assigns its 100 attendings in medicine to four teams, called the Blue, Red, Green, and Gold Firms. An intern spending March on the Red Firm would take care of patients under the supervision of the 25 attendings on that firm.

3. Each patient is assigned to a specific intern or student on a medical team. Thus, the patient is also described as belonging to the team. Services relating to any of the functions described previously, including those of the house staff, nurses, social workers, and so on, are provided by members of the team.
4. The typical student is responsible for 2 to 10 patients. An intern is responsible for 5 to 20 patients.
5. Issues of night coverage, holiday coverage, and other types of helping out are usually organized within the team.

CHAPTER 2

Ambulatory Settings

Ambulatory Medicine: General Principles

1. Medical education is turning increasingly to ambulatory settings. *Ambulatory settings* are those in which the patient has not been admitted to an acute-care hospital. There are numerous types of outpatient practice sites, including hospital clinics, neighborhood health centers, private offices, emergency departments, and urgent care centers.
2. Ambulatory medicine differs from inpatient medicine in several key ways.
   - An ambulatory patient is less likely to come with a preattached diagnosis for the presenting complaint. In the hospital, a patient with known Goodpasture's syndrome might be admitted because of hemoptysis. In the ambulatory setting, you will have to decide whether the patient who is coughing blood has Goodpasture's or something else.
   - The range of pathology is different. Ambulatory patients are, on average, not as sick as hospitalized patients. However, they do present with problems rarely seen in the hospital setting. Some of these are too minor to require hospitalization: sprains, exanthems, localized infections, and the like. Others represent the new onset of major problems: chest pain, a breast nodule, an acute

abdomen, stroke, and others. Others still are not yet fully differentiated: pluripotential symptoms, if you will, such as weight loss, fatigue, or lymphadenopathy.

- Arriving at a precise diagnosis is sometimes less important for outpatients. For conditions such as viral syndrome and musculoskeletal chest pain, it often suffices to judge that the illness is minor and self-limited, liable to improve without strenuous intervention.
- Patients expect evaluation and treatment in a limited period of time, ranging from several minutes to a few hours. This places boundaries around the interaction. Neither lengthy deliberation, nor protracted evaluations by multiple examiners, is generally possible. Punctuality and careful attention to time constraints are crucial.
- The patient typically leaves before results from most tests are available. The clinician must often make important decisions based on an incomplete database.
- Immediate consultation with specialty and subspecialty experts is not widely used.
- Telephone and written communication between the doctor and the patient plays an important role.
- The doctor-patient relation is often protracted. A patient who undergoes cardiac catheterization may never see the invasive cardiologist except on the day of the procedure, or a day before or after. Visits to the clinical cardiologist, on the other hand, may occur every 4 months for 20 years.
- Serial evaluations are often spaced weeks or months apart. The time interval needed for assessing the evolution of an illness, or the response to therapy, is longer than in the hospital.

- Two issues become more prominent for outpatients: compliance and cost to the patient. In the hospital, the medication you order is administered by a nurse to the patient. It does not matter to the patient whether you order penicillin or "Cef-blast-em-all." In the ambulatory setting, the medication you prescribe must be purchased, self-administered according to a schedule, and often refilled by the patient. Any of these steps can go awry.

3. For a student or a house officer, the sequence on an ambulatory encounter is as follows. The student or house officer usually interviews and examines the patient and then presents the case to a supervising physician, generally an attending. These two discuss the case; the attending will often examine the patient as well, and a plan is developed. The assessment and plan are then presented to the patient, and a course of action is undertaken.

   Supervision in ambulatory sites is usually immediate. As the clinician-learner becomes more skilled, he or she assumes more independence in patient care, requiring less intense supervision.
4. Preventive medicine and health screening are *major* ambulatory themes. The typical hospital strategy of addressing the patient's clinical problems, and formulating an assessment and plan, is essentially reactive. While this is an indispensible function in the ambulatory setting as well, there the clinician must also assume a proactive stance in disease prevention and health promotion. Crucial areas include:
   - Immunization
   - Discussion of the impact of behavior and lifestyle on disease (risk factors) and on health (health maintenance)
   - Screening for conditions such as diabetes, hypertension, lipid disorders, malignancy, etc.

Hospital Clinics

1. Most clinical services in the hospital also operate ambulatory clinics. These may be physically located in the hospital, or elsewhere as freestanding enterprises. Their purposes are to provide care within the specialty domain to ambulatory patients and to provide educational sites for students and house officers.

   The hospital clinic is the direct descendant of the dispensary, an area attached to the early hospital, the purpose of which was to provide care at free or reduced cost to indigent members of the surrounding neighborhoods. The dispensaries typically saw large numbers of patients in a short amount of time, with low numbers of physicians, staff, and amenities. Some of these features are still found in today's clinics.

   The term *clinic* is not rigorously defined, but it generally refers to an area of ambulatory care for stable outpatients. The term may also refer to a clinical function, regardless of site; this is especially true of a highly specialized service, such as the spina bifida clinic. Some patients assume that clinics are by definition designed for the poor, with scanty continuity of care; this is not the case.
2. An ambulatory clinic may be devoted to a general field, such as general pediatrics, or to a subspecialty, such as otorhinolaryngology. Clinics may share a single practice site, so that the same set of exam rooms may serve as the dermatology clinic on Thursday and the neurology clinic on Friday.
3. In traditional residency programs, house officers spend one half-day per week, or sometimes more, in an ambulatory clinic. This time for ambulatory practice is likely to increase in the near future. In

most instances, the house officer develops a panel of patients who identify him or her as their doctor. In each clinic session, the house officer sees new and/or established patients, usually by appointment. Each time the patient requires care, he or she sees the same resident, if at all possible; this provides a high degree of continuity of care. In some training programs, patients see whichever resident is available; this does not allow for continuity.

In many programs, residents spend blocks of time, lasting several weeks, entirely in ambulatory clinical experiences.

Residents and students can maintain continuity of care by arranging outpatient visits with their hospitalized patients after discharge. By the same principle, you should attempt to follow patients you have seen in the clinic if they are admitted to the hospital.

4. While many hospital clinics are staffed primarily by residents, other providers such as attendings, nurse-practitioners, and physician assistants may also be seeing patients there. Many clinics are multidisciplinary and provide services by physicians, nurses, social workers, and others.
5. When you follow a patient for longitudinal ambulatory care, you will want to set up one extended visit annually for a comprehensive health evaluation. This is a good way to perform a complete physical examination and to address preventive and screening interventions.
6. One distinguishing feature of hospital clinics is their strong commitment to teaching. Faculty members serve both as supervisors and as teachers; teaching is an intrinsic responsibility, not a superfluous assignment. At the same time, clinic patients usually understand that they are receiving care from trainees, under expert supervision.

Neighborhood Health Centers

1. Neighborhood health centers are offices set up in residential communities. They often focus on providing care to underserved populations, such as the indigent, low wage earners, the elderly, and minority groups. They are typically structured as multispecialty group practices, emphasizing primary care. Many are not-for-profit organizations, and many receive external financial support from government agencies or charitable grants.
2. Students and residents may see patients at neighborhood health centers, on either an interim or a long-term basis. The primary purpose of the centers is to provide care; teaching functions are secondary. However, they can provide clinicians with opportunities for community outreach, for seeing diverse types of patients, and for evaluating clinical problems that have not been divided according to specialty area. Patients will often be grateful to see medical students and residents, who wear the mantle of the university and who can contribute significantly to the amount and quality of care being delivered.

Physician Offices

1. Two traditional practice formats are the solo practice and the group practice. In a *solo practice*, an individual practitioner sees patients, collects fees, and pays for overhead and staffing. Whatever revenue is left constitutes the physician's income. In *group practices*, two or more physicians share these responsibilities and share revenues. In a third form of practice, physicians are employed by a corporation to perform medical services; in this format, income is based on a salary plus additional payments for seeing larger numbers of patients.

Medical professionals are turning increasingly to larger and larger group practices as a strategy for reducing costs, sharing overhead, and spreading out such responsibilities as off-hours call, vacation coverage, and so forth.

2. There is a growing trend to assign students and residents to office practice sites. This promises to expand further the types of patients the clinician encounters, although there are formidable obstacles. The office is not designed for teaching purposes; the learners are guests. Trainees slow the flow of patients, reducing income to the practice. The patients usually assume that they will see their accustomed physician and may be surprised to see a student or resident. Further, the presence of a trainee may disrupt to some extent the personal relation between the doctor and the patient. Nonetheless, many medical schools and residency programs are exploring new ways to bring students to offices for educationally meaningful experiences.

The Emergency Department

1. The emergency department is located within the hospital and serves patients who identify themselves as having medical emergencies. Patients who present to the emergency department are evaluated and then either admitted to the hospital, or treated and discharged.
2. The first evaluation occurs in the triage area, in which a member of the medical staff—usually a nurse—assesses the severity and the acuity of the patient's complaint. Patients who are deemed severely or acutely ill are then sent immediately to physicians for evaluation. Patients who are deemed less ill take second priority. Many hospitals have urgent care centers to which patients are referred if their illnesses do not appear to require emergency

services. For students and residents, the urgent care center is an opportunity to care for musculoskeletal injuries, lacerations, minor infections, dermatologic problems, etc.

3. The physician role may be played by residents, attendings, nurse-practitioners, or physician assistants. The clinician is expected to see patients promptly, again prioritizing according to severity and acuity of illness as well as by the patient's time of arrival. He or she will evaluate the patient, then present the case to an attending, and then institute a management plan.
4. Students also assume the physician role. The attending or resident will usually identify which patients are most appropriate for the student; the rest of the evaluation proceeds as for residents.
5. Emergency medicine is distinguished not only by the pressing nature of serious illness, but also by a reliance on practice protocols. The role of the emergency physician is often not to make a certain diagnosis, but rather to stabilize the immediate situation and to refer to other practitioners for definitive care. "Through-put" is critically important; a bottled-up emergency department cannot meet the needs of newly arriving patients.

The Telephone

1. In ambulatory medicine, the telephone has become an essential instrument for doctor-patient communication. It is used for the initial assessment of symptoms, for recommending therapy, for assessing patient progress, and for reporting laboratory data.
2. For all telephone calls with patients, it is essential to:
   - Identify yourself and your function to the patient
   - Keep a written record, including the patient's name, the date and time, and your name

- Record the substance of the conversation
- Sign your record and ensure that it is entered into the medical record
- Review the call with a supervising physician and obtain his or her countersignature

3. For calls related to the assessment of a medical complaint, additional points are to:
   - Identify the chief complaint and pertinent features of the history
   - Note the patient's medical conditions, medications, and drug allergies, if the patient's chart is not directly at hand
   - Record your assessment and plan
   - Discuss the assessment and plan with the supervising physician, if necessary, before communicating it to the patient, which frequently requires that you call the patient back
   - Recommend that the patient be evaluated at once in an emergency department, if his or her condition could be severe or life threatening
4. For calls in which you recommend therapy, it is necessary to:
   - Explain exactly what you are recommending
   - Describe medications precisely, including their name, dose, and frequency of administration
   - Discuss possible adverse reactions
   - Make contingency plans (e.g., "If the pain gets worse, call me back.")
5. For calls relating to the evaluation of a patient's progress, it is important to:
   - Ask specifically about the cardinal features of the illness (e.g., if on Monday you begin oral antibiotics for a patient with pneumonia, on Tuesday you will want to call and ask specifically about fever, cough, dyspnea, and sputum.)
   - Ask whether adverse reactions have occurred
6. For calls in which you relate laboratory data, it is advisable to:

- Explain not only what the test results are, but also what they mean (e.g., "Your creatinine has increased" is not so meaningful to most patients as "Your kidney function appears to be getting worse.")
- Make a plan for responses to abnormal results

7. Interns and residents, but not students, can telephone prescriptions to pharmacies. As in a written prescription, you should describe the name of the medication, the tablet or capsule size, the amount to be dispensed, how the medication is to be taken, whether generic substitution is permitted, and whether refills are permitted. The pharmacist may ask for the prescriber's address, telephone number, medical license number, and occasionally the Drug Enforcement Administration number. Controlled substances, however, cannot usually be prescribed by telephone.
8. Evaluation by telephone is less certain than evaluation by face-to-face interviewing and examination. However, face-to-face evaluation is often not necessary. You should feel completely comfortable in assessing and treating minor infections, gastrointestinal complaints, injuries, and other ailments. For patients with more serious illnesses, but who are essentially stable, small adjustments in therapy are also legitimate.

   If you are in doubt, or if the patient's condition sounds significantly abnormal or changed, it is best to recommend that he or she be seen by a physician.
9. Courtesy, promptness, rationality, and concern are as important on the telephone as in the office.

CHAPTER 3

Rounds

Rounds Explained

1. *Rounds* refers to the physician's visits to patients. In one sense of the term, a physician seeing patients in the hospital is said to be making rounds. In another sense, rounds are the collective activities of physicians, students, and other staff members—usually in seeing patients, but also in conferring or learning.

   Rounds are thus the main interaction between doctors and (hospitalized) patients, and among doctors.
2. The several types of rounds are Morning Rounds, Work Rounds, Attending Rounds, "Chart Rounds," Sign-Out Rounds, and Grand Rounds.

Morning Rounds

1. Morning Rounds are usually the first collective activity of the day. The purpose of Morning Rounds is for the members of the health-care team to share information and plans.
2. What happens on Morning Rounds:
   - New admissions are presented. Each new case should take 5 to 10 minutes.
   - Major new problems are reviewed.

- Major updates (major test results, diagnostic findings, etc.) are discussed.
- The residents teach. Residents are the main teachers on Morning Rounds. They have the responsibility of reviewing the current literature regarding clinical issues that arise in the course of patient care. They may make a 5-minute presentation on such an issue. They may also ask you to prepare a brief presentation, or you may offer to present the results of your own reading—if it would be of general interest to the group. For example, if your patient has hyperparathyroidism, you will want to read up on the differential diagnosis and management options for this problem—and you may be asked to share your findings with the group.

3. It is your responsibility to come to rounds prepared. This means that you:
   - Have seen your patients and examined them, before rounds
   - Know their vital signs
   - Know the results of their diagnostic tests
   - Know the input from the attending physician, consultants, nurses, etc.
   - Have formulated a plan for their care
   - Are ready to present any new admissions
4. Morning Rounds may take place in a conference room, nurses station, patient lounge, or corridor. As always, patient *confidentiality* carries the utmost importance. Patient discussions must not take place within earshot of passersby. If visitors approach, pause until they have passed.
5. Morning Rounds are usually run by one (or more) of the residents. They may begin as early as 5:30 AM on some surgical services or as late as 8:00 AM on some specialized services. They generally last 30 to 60 minutes.

Work Rounds

1. Generally Work Rounds directly follow Morning Rounds. The purpose of Work Rounds is for the team as a group, or subgroup, to see each patient. Each member of the team will therefore be familiar with the major clinical issues for each patient. Morning Rounds and Work Rounds are sometimes combined into a single event, going by either name. This combined event is especially common on weekends and holidays.
2. What happens on Work Rounds:
   - Each patient is interviewed and examined. Each member of the team should examine important areas. For example, in a patient with congestive heart failure, each student, intern, and resident should auscultate the lungs.
   - The diagnostic process, so far, is reviewed with the patient.
   - Plans for further testing, procedures, treatment, and discharge are reviewed with the patient.

   Keeping the patient informed is crucial. Patients are justifiably upset when they are whisked off to a test that they've never heard of, or when they first learn on Tuesday night that they will be discharged on Wednesday.

   Nurses or social worker may participate. A faculty member may be present to augment the educational process, or to supervise.
3. It is your responsibility to take the lead with your patients. You should be the first to greet the patient, to ask how he/she is feeling, and to perform an examination. This may recap, to a certain extent, the interaction that occurred before Morning Rounds.

   It is crucial that you be the one to take charge regarding your patients. If you hold back and stay at the back of the crowd, someone else is likely to become impatient and run the show.

4. Work Rounds are for work. Practical diagnostic and management questions are entirely appropriate. However, more general, academic questions are better left to other occasions.

Attending Rounds

1. Attending Rounds are small teaching conferences in which the team meets with a faculty member. Their purpose is to learn from the cases on the service.
2. What happens in Attending Rounds:
   - The group usually meets in a conference room or lounge.
   - A student or intern presents a case. Remember that the goal is to use the case as a springboard for discussion, not to demonstrate how many details you elicited.
   - The group then discusses the educational issues in the case. These might include basic science points, differential diagnosis, clinical management, or recent research.
   - The group may see the patient together to review points in the history or physical examination.
   - One or two cases are usually discussed. Sessions usually last 30 to 60 minutes and may occur every 1 to 7 days.
3. It is your responsibility to:
   - Present a case.
   - Know the clinicial issues especially well for a case you are presenting.
   - Bring x-rays, histologic slides, or other materials, if appropriate.
   - Learn.
   - Be mindful of the learning needs and prerogatives of the other members of the team.

- Ask the patient, in advance, if he or she would mind being seen by a somewhat larger group than usual. Most patients will agree, if they are given advance notice and an opportunity to ask questions.

"Chart Rounds"

1. Chart Rounds exist at some hospitals. Their purpose is for the resident to review the day's events for each patient with the student and/or intern caring for the patient.
2. What happens at Chart Rounds:
   - The resident meets with the student and/or intern, usually at the nursing station, and usually in the afternoon.
   - Events, input from other caregivers, findings, and lab results from the day are reviewed.
   - Ongoing plans are formulated and revised.
3. Your responsibilities include:
   - Gathering results from laboratory tests, x-rays, biopsies, etc.
   - Interpreting these results.
   - Making a plan. Generally, you should take the initiative in planning your patient's evaluation and care. The resident will review your decisions with you and explain reasons for agreement or disagreement. This active role is better than waiting passively to be told what to do; you did not go to medical school to become a scribe or a "gofer."

Sign-Out Rounds

1. Sign-Out Rounds take place at the end of the day, before team members leave the hospital. Their purpose is to transmit the most vital information regarding patients to the on-call team.

2. What happens at Sign-Out Rounds:
   - You will meet with the person on call for the evening.
   - You will make an organized list that tells, for each of your patients:
     - Major diagnoses and problems
     - Major medications
     - Allergies
     - Severity of illness
     - *Is there anything to do or check that evening?*

       Examples:

       - "Draw CBC at 10 PM."
       - "Listen to lungs after blood transfusion; if rales, give furosemide 40 mg IVP."
     - Major contingency plans

       Examples:

       - "If Hgb <9.0, call surgery resident to evalu ate for possible surgery tonight."
       - "If recurrence of chest pain, start heparin IV."
     - *Resuscitation status* (whether do-not-resuscitate [DNR] or not)
     - Attending physician
   - You will review the list verbally with the on-call person.
3. It is your responsibility to:
   - Make your sign-out list accurate, organized, and concise.
   - Spell out the likely "what-if" scenarios as carefully as possible. You have had opportunity to reflect on your patient's overall situation; the on-call person has not.
   - *Request only essential actions* from the on-call person. Asking the on-call person to check breath sounds on an asthmatic is a good idea; asking him or her to replace an IV that just fell out is not.

- Minimize the number of lab tests whose values will become available during the evening or night. Try, as much as possible, to obtain lab results before you leave for the evening. This is especially true for an arterial blood gas; if you draw one, don't go home until you know, and have responded to, the result.
- Be very clear regarding DNR status.

4. If you are the on-call person, you want to be sure that you understand each of these issues for each patient. If the sign-out list is unclear, talk with your colleague to clarify each point.

Grand Rounds

Grand Rounds used to mean that a renowned professor would see a patient *en masse* with the collected faculty and students. It has kept that name, out of respect for a grand old tradition, but now refers to a lecture, often by a visiting speaker of some type.

"Roundsmanship"

1. The purposes of the various forms of rounds are to evaluate patients, relate patient information, and learn. It is not a time to show off, demonstrate your "brilliance," or compete.
2. Medical rounds have been called "the last one-room schoolhouse." This means that learners of varying levels of expertise, ranging from early clinical students to house officers to faculty members, are trying to learn at the same time, in the same place. Each member of the team can, and should, learn from the experience. Each should remember the learning needs of everyone else.
3. Rounds tend *not* to work if:
   - Someone monopolizes the discussion.

- Someone focuses the entire discussion to his or her personal level. This bores those with more experience, and stifles those with less.
- Someone transmits facts without considering if others are likely to receive the transmission, or to benefit from it.

Is it right, is it even prudence ,
To bore thyself, and bore the students?
—Goethe, Faust. Transl. Walter Kaufmann

4. Manuals and how-to's on Rounds are usually dedicated to making you look smart. You don't need to look smart. You do need to *be* smart, to be respectful of others, to care for your patients, and to learn.

CHAPTER 4

Writing Notes

General Principles

1. Medical notes serve several functions:
   - They record the *history* and *physical examination*, both on admission and on a daily basis.
   - They record data from *laboratory tests*.
   - They document the on-going *interpretation* of findings.
   - They document the *plan* for testing and care.
   - They record *events*: procedures, operations, and other happenings.
   - They provide a vehicle for communication among doctors and other caregivers.
   - They record recommendations from consultants.
   - They record results of discussions with patients or families, including issues of consent, agreement with the care plan, advance directives, and resuscitation wishes.
   - They are a permanent legal record of a patient's care.
2. Medical students and interns have an especially important role in the medical chart. They are usually responsible for:
   - Documenting the history, physical examination, and lab data for each day of hospitalization.
   - Recording results of tests, which should be entered as soon as they are available. If your patient

has a computed tomography [CT] scan on Tuesday, you should see the scan and record its results by Wednesday at the latest.

- Interpreting results. It is not enough to transcribe what someone else has said; you should show that you understand what's happening and have thought about it.
- Showing that all salient points of a case have been addressed. This means that you must read what everyone has said and can put together diverse points of view. If the patient has a new symptom, if the hemoglobin falls, if the nurse says that the patient is confused at night, if the physical therapist says that the patient can't walk—you must address each point, interpret it, and make a plan.

> 1. Address each point.
> 2. Interpret it.
> 3. Make a plan.

3. The note, like the entire medical chart, is a legal record. Anything that anyone writes is subject to review. This has several implications:
   - Be sure to follow the rules listed in #4, the next section.
   - Document all pertinent facts.
   - Make sure that all opinions voiced in the chart are well-founded and relevant. Opinion is a necessary part of medical practice. Opinions entered into the medical record, however, should be substantiated. Speculation and guesswork do not belong in the chart.
   - The chart is not the proper place for disputes. You may think that the renal consultant is an imbecile, but you should address her views with objectivity and respect.
   - A new event often has implications for action. A new fever generally implies some sort of diagnos-

tic evaluation, such as history, physical exam, chest x-ray (CXR), urinalysis, etc. If you record the event, you should also record what you did about it.

- Anything that might be controversial should be reviewed with a supervising physician, such as your resident, before you enter it into the record.

4. A few rules:
   - All notes must be dated and timed.
   - Identify who you are and in what capacity you are writing the note, for example, Med Student Progress Note; MS Vascular Surgery Consult.
   - Sign all notes, followed by your "rank": MS 3, MS 4, MD.
   - All student and intern notes must be countersigned. It is your responsibility to see that your notes are countersigned.
5. **Language.** The aim is to be precise and succinct. When medical terms are more accurate than common English, use them. "Epigastric pain" is more accurate than "stomach pain," and "dyspnea" is good shorthand for "shortness of breath." However, *common English is often just fine.* "Leg" is better than "lower extremity."

   It is important to be neither more precise, nor less, than the patient's account allows. If the patient complains of dizziness, you will try to pin down which of the several senses of the word she means: vertigo, presyncope, altered balance, etc. If she cannot specify exactly what she means, it is better to label the issue as "dizziness" than to force her symptom into your category.
6. **Quantification.** Most symptoms and findings can be quantified on a scale of mild-moderate-severe. Some have other conventional scales. For example:
   - *Chest pain*: scale 1 (very slight) to 10 (worst I ever felt in my life)

- *Heart murmur*: scale 1 (barely audible) to 6 (heard without a stethoscope)
- *Peripheral edema*: scale 1 (slight) to 4 (severe)
- *Peripheral pulses*: scale 1+ (decreased but palpable) to 4+ (bounding) (The plus signs have no particular meaning.)

The term *trace* is sometimes used to describe the quantity "more than zero but less than one."

These scales are relative. By asking more experienced physicians how they would grade a particular finding, you can set your own parameters.

7. The results of certain common blood tests are often portrayed using stick figures.
   - Complete blood count (CBC)

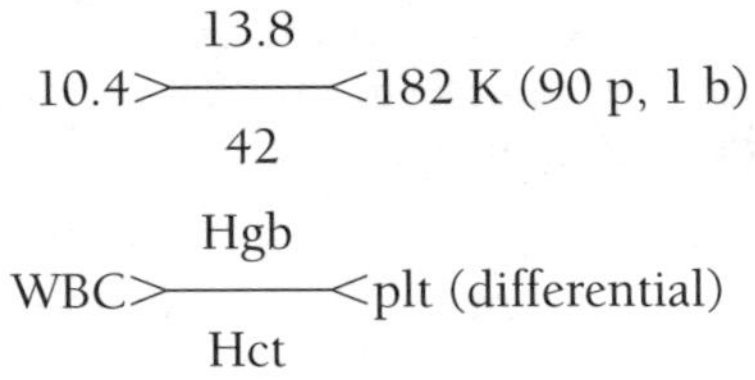

```
           13.8
  10.4>───────────<182 K (90 p, 1 b)
            42

            Hgb
   WBC>───────────<plt (differential)
            Hct
```

   - Abbreviations
     - Hgb = hemoglobin
     - Hct = hematocrit
     - WBC = white blood cell count
     - plt = platelets
     - p = polymorphonucleocytes
     - b = bands
     - l = lymphocytes
     - m = monocytes
     - K = thousand
   - Electrolytes, renal function, glucose

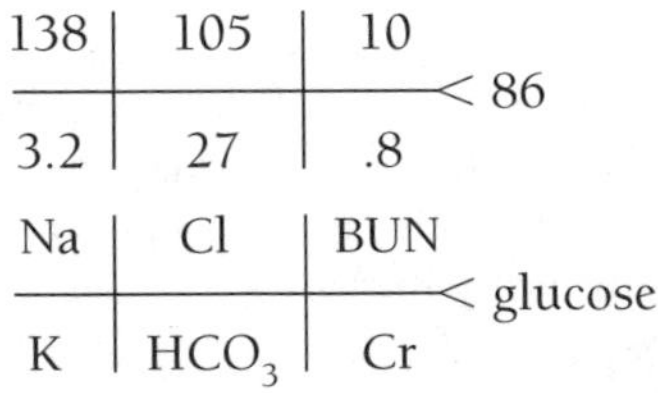

```
 138 |  105  |  10
─────┼───────┼──────< 86
 3.2 |  27   |  .8

 Na  |  Cl   | BUN
─────┼───────┼──────< glucose
  K  | HCO3  |  Cr
```

- Abbreviations
  Na = sodium
  K = potassium
  Cl = chloride
  HCO_3 = bicarbonate
  BUN = blood urea nitrogen
  Cr = creatinine

8. Do's and Don'ts of Notes

Do

- Record *vital signs* daily.
  The temperature is best recorded as Tmax, the maximum temperature during the previous 24 hours.
  The blood pressure, heart rate, and respiratory rate are best recorded in terms of their ranges during the previous 24 hours.
  Body weight is measured and recorded on admission and thereafter as often as clinically indicated. A patient with congestive heart failure, for example, should be weighed daily. Most patients should be weighed once or twice a week.
- *Record and interpret all significant new events.*
- Record *test results* as they become available. If Monday's CBC isn't complete when you write Monday's note, write "CBC pending" and enter the results later on Monday, as an addendum.
- If a new event or finding occurs, record it promptly.
- *Highlight significant findings.*
- Keep a daily log of outstanding tests:
  - Tests that have been ordered but not yet performed
  - Tests that have been performed but for which results are not available
- Write medications and doses frequently—perhaps daily. Check what you think the patient is receiving against the nurse's records (sometimes called the *Medex*), which document what the patient is

actually receiving. There are a number of reasons to check this record:

- The nurse might withhold a dose, if he or she thought it could be harmful.
- The patient may have been unable to take a dose.
- The patient may have refused a dose.
- The medication or dose might have been transcribed incorrectly.
- Someone else might have ordered a new drug, or discontinued a drug.
- You might have forgotten to discontinue a drug that you intended to stop.

- Track antibiotics. "Piperacillin day 4/7" means that the patient is on day 4 of a planned 7-day course.
- Track the number of days after a major event; for example, "postop day 3" or "CCU day 17."
- Talk to the nurses and read their notes.
- Outline the plan for further care each day.
- If you carry a beeper, write its number after your signature.
- Make your own plan and show your reasoning. You are not a robot, not a transparent scribe, and not a dope.
- Document important discussions with the patient or the family.
- If you have an idea that you're not sure of, you can introduce it into the record by writing something like the following: *"Consider liver biopsy; will discuss with Dr. Saugerties."*
- Write in black ink. Dark blue ink is sometimes acceptable. Red ink may be used for procedure notes and surgical notes.

Don't

- Don't write "AF VSS"—never, nohow. This is sometimes used as shorthand for "afebrile, vital signs stable." It has no informational content whatsoever.

- Don't record new events without offering an interpretation. Don't report a new fever without adding "Fever" to the problem list and analyzing both what you think is happening and what you plan to do about it.
- Don't write that a lab test is "Pending" if the result should be available.
- Don't leave blank spaces, or blank stick figures, in the note. It is illegal to back-enter data into a note. This amounts to falsifying the record.
- Don't write "stable" unless the patient is truly stable; for example, 4 days after an uncomplicated cholecystectomy.
- Don't criticize others in the chart.
- Don't enter opinions that are unsubstantiated.
- Don't write long summaries every day.
- Don't copy passages from textbooks or articles. Controversial points can be supported with references.

Admission Notes

1. The purpose of the admission note is to provide a complete register of both the present illness and the patient's overall health.
2. Admission notes are written according to the SOAP format.

Subjective. *What the Patient Says*
Record the patient's description of symptoms and his or her sense of improvement or worsening.

Objective. *What Has Been Found About the Patient*
Record your physical examination.
Then list lab tests with results.

Then list lab tests for which results are still pending.

Assessment. *Your Interpretation*

Organize a list of the salient clinical issues, the problem list (see Chapter 14).

Record what you think is going on for each issue.

Plan

What are you going to do about it?

3. The admission note follows a standard sequence.

Format for the Admission Note

1. History
   a. Chief Complaint
   b. History of the Present Illness
   c. Past Medical History
   d. Social History
   e. Family History
   f. Review of Systems
2. Physical Examination
3. Laboratory Data
4. Summary
5. Assessment
6. Plan

4. **Chief Complaint.** The chief complaint should list the patient's age, gender, history of major illnesses, and the immediate issue at hand.

Examples

Ms. Gutz is a 46-year-old woman with rheumatoid arthritis who is admitted because of fever and abdominal pain for 2 days.

Bart Reglar is a 19-year-old man with diabetes mellitus who was referred from his physician's office because of altered mental status.

Miles Gloriosus is a 39-year-old man, previously well, who came to the emergency room stating, "I couldn't breathe," for 30 min.

The chief complaint is like a headline and should contain crucial news only. It does not need to include less important data, such as the number of hospital admissions. Biographic information, such as occupation and marital status, are *ordinarily* best left for the Social History. Race and ethnicity should be addressed consistently. If you identify race or ethnicity for minority populations, you should identify them for majority populations as well. Otherwise, the implication is that one ethnicity is normal and that all others need to be specified.

The chief complaint should be stated in the most accurate possible terms. This *might* be the patient's own words, but need not be.

5. **History of the Present Illness (HPI).** The HPI should start at the beginning of the *presenting* illness, not at the beginning of all illness.

Example

> The patient first noted right leg pain 7 mo ago, when she developed cramping in the calf after walking a quarter mile. Symptoms were relieved in <5 min with rest. . . .

Previous medical conditions, if potentially relevant to the presenting illness, should be summarized in the first sentence.

Examples

> The patient had Dukes A colon carcinoma, resected 3 yr ago, but has had no subsequent abdominal symptoms until yesterday, when he developed nausea, vomiting, and abdominal pain. . . .

> The patient has had end-stage renal disease due to polycystic kidneys, treated with peritoneal dialysis for 2 yr, but was otherwise well until 2 days ago, when he noted loss of vision in his left eye for 20 min. . . .

You should specify pertinent positive and negative features of the history.

Examples

> The pain was accompanied by dyspnea and lightheadedness but not by nausea, vomiting, diaphoresis, or radiation.

> Headache was worse when lying down and relieved by sitting up; there was no fever, stiff neck, or photophobia.

The last sentence of the HPI should be a review of systems for the organ system that seems responsible for the patient's acute illness.

Example

> *For a male patient admitted with acute urinary retention*: He reports nocturia 2×/night for 1 year and occasional hesitancy but denies dysuria, discharge, hematuria, urinary tract infections, nephrolithiasis, or known kidney disease.

6. **Past Medical History (PMH).** The PMH follows a set format.
   a. Medical Illnesses
   b. Surgical Illnesses
   c. Psychiatric Illnesses
   d. Medications
   e. Allergies to Medications
   f. Smoking, Alcohol, and Recreational Drug Use (sometimes placed in Social History instead)
   g. Screen for Possible Exposures to HIV (transfusion, intravenous drug use, multiple sexual partners)
7. **Social History.** The Social History also follows a format.
   a. *Occupation* (present or former). Don't assume that the elderly or the disabled are necessarily unemployed.

b. *Marital status.*
c. *Sexual orientation and practices.* Use your judgment here. Circumstances greatly affect how complete a sexual history should be. Someone with fever and lymphadenopathy, or with secondary amenorrhea, should have a detailed sexual history. For an 89-year-old admitted for cataract resection, this is less pertinent—perhaps completely irrelevant.

8. **Family History.** Again, completeness should vary according to circumstances. A complete genealogy is not necessary for a patient admitted for cataract surgery. A few screening questions related to family history of heart disease, cancer, diabetes, or eye disease are more to the point.

   For some conditions, a detailed family history is particularly important. These include congenital abnormalities, cancer, coronary artery disease, diabetes, lipid disorders, inflammatory bowel disease, kidney disease, menstrual abnormalities, and others.

9. **Review of Systems (ROS).** The ROS can be completed as a sort of checklist. Most truly pertinent issues will be entered into the Past Medical History.

   A sample is listed in the example at the end of the chapter.

10. **Physical Examination.** For an admission note, the complete physical examination should be recorded.
    - In general, use the example at the end of the chapter as a template.
    - Highlight important findings.

11. **Laboratory Data.** A certain set of laboratory data are obtained on admission for virtually all new patients. These include the following, which should be entered into the admission note:
    - Complete blood count (CBC)
    - Electrolytes, renal parameters, glucose (SMA 7)

(This sometimes includes a full biochemistry panel.)
- Urinalysis (UA)
- Electrocardiogram (EKG)
- X-rays

Other studies should of course be recorded if they have been performed.

12. **Summary.** This is your chance to distill the case down to its absolute essence. As a rough guideline, you should devote a single sentence to each category of the history, to the physical examination, and to lab data.

Example

> In summary, Mr. Gonasch is a 24-year-old man with steroid-dependent asthma who is admitted because of right hip pain for 3 days. The past history is notable for asthma, requiring prednisone 10–30 mg daily for 3 mo, and for viral meningitis at age 6. Physical exam is notable for a clear chest, for moderate tenderness on deep palpation of the hip anteriorly, and for moderate pain with internal rotation of the hip. Lab data are notable for normal CBC and glucose 146. Hip x-ray is normal; bone scan demonstrates increased uptake in the hip.

13. **Assessment.** The overall design of the assessment is to list the major problems at hand, and then to write what you think the major issues in differential diagnosis are. You should show your reasoning.

Example

> 1. Hip pain. Differential diagnosis of patient's acute hip pain includes avascular necrosis, septic arthritis, gonococcal arthritis, and fracture. Avascular necrosis is suggested by the history of steroid use and by the bone scan finding. Septic arthritis would be likely

to have fever; this might however be blunted by steroid use. There is no history of gonococcus exposure, although this should always be considered. Fracture is not evident on plain films; they could however miss an early, small, nondisplaced fracture.

2. Hyperglycemia. Mild increased glucose probably due to glucocorticoid use combined with acute stress reaction.
3. Asthma. Stable at present. Chronic steroid use mandates monitoring for signs of adrenal insufficiency.

There are three formats for the assessment and plan.

- Each problem, then a plan for each problem.

Example

1. Hip pain discussion
   Plan for hip pain
2. Hyperglycemia discussion
   Plan for hyperglycemia
3. Discussion of other problems
   Plans for other problems

- All the problems, then all the plans.

Example

1. Hip pain discussion
2. Hyperglycemia discussion
3. Discussion of other problems

1. Plan for hip pain
2. Plan for hyperglycemia
3. Plan for other problems

This is my choice for most cases. It identifies the plan in a separate place, so that everyone sees what you think should be done.

- For complex, multisystem diseases, it is best to consider each organ system separately. This is a good system for notes in intensive care.

Example

Pulmonary: Pt severely dyspneic on admission with pulmonary edema on chest x-ray and arterial blood gas 7.25/pCO_2 28/PO_2 44/76% O_2 saturation. Pt now intubated on Assist Control at 18 breaths/min with FiO_2 50%, Tidal volume 750 mL, PEEP 5 cm; ABG 7.28/32/120/94%. Pattern of pulmonary edema with respiratory acidosis suggests sepsis with ARDS.

Cardiac: Initial BP 94/68, HR 116, with S_4 gallop but no jugular venous distention. Right heart catheter indicated pulmonary capillary wedge pressure 15 cm, implying noncardiogenic pulmonary edema.

GI: ALT and AST elevated at 112 and 98 respectively. DDx includes shock liver, hepatitis, or drug effect.

Renal: Urine output 30–40 mL/hr with creatinine 1.8 and few granular casts on urinalysis. Findings indicate. . .

Hematology:

Infectious diseases:

Neurology:

14. **Plan.** This is your place to make a plan of action for each problem. As mentioned above, plans can be listed after each problem individually, or after the entire assessment.

Example

Plan

1. Joint aspiration under fluoroscopic guidance. Fluid to be sent for cell count, Gram's stain, and culture.
2. If organisms seen on Gram's stain → intravenous antibiotics.

3. Bed rest.
4. Analgesia with codeine 30 mg q6h prn.
5. Check fingerstick glucose qid.
6. Continue prednisone 30 mg qd.
7. If signs of hypotension or unexplained clinical deterioration occur, consider adrenal insufficiency and treat with hydrocortisone 100 mg IVSS q8h.

Contingency plans (if → then), such as #2 and #7 in the preceding list, are a good idea and help to demonstrate your thought process. They also help guide another's response, if you're not available.

Progress Notes

1. The purpose of progress notes is to provide a daily account of the major features of the patient's illness and treatment. Every patient has a progress note on every day, and you will write the progress note for each of your patients.
2. Progress notes are written according to the *SOAP* format. Examples appear at the end of this chapter.
3. The three formats for organizing the assessment and plan, described under Admission Notes, are equally pertinent in the Progress Note.
4. For the assessment and plan sections of the Progress Note, it is helpful to keep a running list of all the problems that have emerged during the hospitalization.

Example

A patient with pyelonephritis has asthma that is well-controlled.

Assessment

1. *Pyelonephritis:* Pt currently afebrile and has no further flank pain. Urine cultures are posi-

tive for *E coli*, sensitive to ampicillin; blood cultures remain negative.
2. *Asthma.* Stable; no wheezing or dyspnea on current regimen.

Plan
1. Change antibiotics to ampicillin 2 g IVSS q4hr.
2. Continue albuterol inhaler.

Update Notes

1. The purpose of update notes is to record new, important events. Update notes are also written according to the *SOAP* format. An example appears at the end of this chapter.
2. You should write an update note:
   - When the patient develops an important new symptom

   Examples: hemoptysis, altered mental status, cold extremity

   - When the patient develops an important new physical finding

   Examples: asymmetric pupillary response, tachypnea

   - When an important new lab result is available

   Examples: positive biopsy, positive blood culture

   - Whenever news occurs that is too important to wait for the next progress note
3. Update notes are especially important when you are covering for another student or physician.

Procedure Notes

The purpose of procedure notes is to document the performance of a procedure.

Format

1. Name of procedure
2. Indication
3. Consent: How obtained, potential complications, content of discussion, patient's agreement
4. Operators: Who did it (This generally means you, plus whoever supervised you.)
5. Anesthesia: Local, general, regional
6. Procedure: What you did
7. Findings (when relevant)
8. Complications

Sample Procedure Note #1

Your patient requires lumbar puncture.

7/24/95 2:30 PM Procedure Note

Procedure: Lumbar puncture.

Indication: Fever, stiff neck.

Consent: Risks and benefits of LP were discussed with patient, including possibility of headache, CSF leak, infection. Patient expresses understanding of these possibilities and agrees to procedure. Signed consent in chart.

Operators: Heberden MS 3, Ponekopf, MD.

Anesthesia: Local.

Procedure: The fundi showed no papilledema. The patient was placed in the lateral decubitus position. The skin was cleansed with povidone solution and draped in the usual sterile fashion. The skin was anesthetized with 1% lidocaine. Using sterile technique, the subdural space was entered without difficulty and 20 mL of clear, colorless fluid was obtained. Patient tolerated procedure well.

Findings: Opening pressure 180 mm. Fluid was sent for cell count, glucose, protein, cytology, Gram's stain, and culture.

Complications: None

Bill Heberden MS 3
HEBERDEN
BP 1234

Sample Procedure Note #2

Your patient, who is severely burned and lethargic, requires a central venous catheter for the administration of hyperalimentation.

7/25/95 4:50 PM Procedure Note

Procedure: Left subclavian vein catheterization.

Indication: Hyperalimentation.

Consent: Risks and benefits of subclavian vein catheterization were discussed with patient's wife, including possibility of pneumothorax, bleeding, or infection. She expresses understanding of these possibilities and agrees to procedure. Signed consent in chart.

Operators: Heberden MS 3, Ponekopf, MD.

Anesthesia: Local.

Procedure: The patient was placed in slight Trendelenburg position. The skin was cleansed with povidone solution and draped in the usual sterile fashion. The skin was anesthetized with 1% lidocaine. Using sterile technique, a triple lumen venous catheter was introduced into the left subclavian vein. Good blood return was demonstrated for each port. Patient tolerated procedure well.

Complications: None. Chest x-ray ordered.

Bill Heberden MS3
HEBERDEN
BP 1234

Surgical Notes

The purpose of surgical notes, also called *operative notes*, is to document the performance of an operation.

Format

1. Name of operation
2. Indication
3. Consent: How obtained, potential complications, content of discussion, patient's agreement
4. Operators: Who did it (include the name of the attending surgeon and assistants)
5. Anesthesia: Local, general, regional (include the name of the anesthesiologist(s))
6. Preoperative diagnosis: The working diagnosis before surgery
7. Surgical diagnosis: The working diagnosis based on surgical findings
8. Procedure: What you did
9. Findings
10. Specimens: What tissue was removed, and what studies it was sent for
11. Estimated blood loss
12. Drains: Type of surgical drains placed, and where
13. Complications
14. Disposition

There will often be two surgical notes, a complete surgical note that is dictated and a brief surgical note that is written in the chart. They are similar in format but different in content, in that the dictated note describes each step of the operation in complete detail. The written note describes the procedure itself in a highly abbreviated fashion, or not at all.

Sample Surgical Note

Your patient has just undergone transurethral resection of the prostate.

10/26/95 6:30 PM Operative Note

Procedure: TURP.

Indication: Urinary retention.

Consent: Risks and benefits of TURP were discussed with patient, including possibility of incontinence, erectile dysfunction, bleeding. Patient expresses understanding of these possibilities and agrees to procedure. Signed consent in chart.

Operators: Dr. Pickelhelm. Assistants Heberden MS 3, Ponekopf, MD.

Anesthesia: Spinal. Dr. Tiefschlaf.

Preoperative Diagnosis: Benign prostatic hypertrophy.

Surgical Diagnosis: Prostatic carcinoma.

Specimens: Chips sent for fresh frozen sections; 2 of 4 sections positive for adenocarcinoma.

Estimated Blood Loss: 250 mL.

Drains: Continuous bladder irrigation via Foley catheter.

Complications: None.

Disposition: Patient was transferred to the recovery room alert, awake and in stable condition.

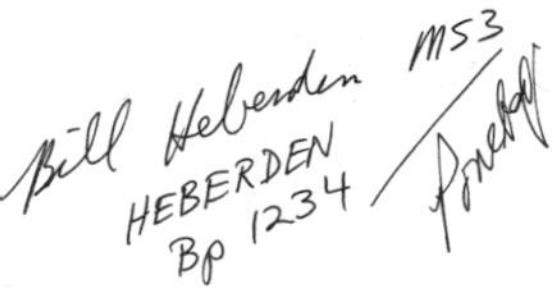

Discharge Notes

The purpose of the discharge note is to document the plans for continued care at the time of discharge from the hospital.

Format

1. Principal Diagnosis
2. Secondary Diagnoses
3. Medications
4. Activity
5. Diet
6. Follow-Up
7. Special Instructions

Sample Discharge Note

Your patient has been hospitalized for acute pyelonephritis.

11/8/95 10:00 AM Discharge Note

Principal Diagnosis: Acute pyelonephritis.

Secondary Diagnoses: Polycystic kidney disease.
Hypertension.

Medications: Amoxicillin 500 mg TID for 7 days.
Enalapril 10 mg QD.
Ortho-Novum 7-7-7, 1 QD.

Activity: Ad lib as tolerated.

Diet: Regular.

Follow-Up: Dr. Gelbwasser 1 wk.

Instructions: Pt instructed to call Dr. Gelbwasser in event of fever, dysuria, or back pain.

Bill Heberden MS3
HEBERDEN
Bp 1234

Outpatient Notes

The purpose of outpatient notes is to document the history, physical examination, assessment, and plan for outpatient visits. Outpatient notes follow the **SOAP** format.

Outpatient notes resemble inpatient admission and progress notes, except that:

- Medications should be listed for every visit.
- Attention should be given not only to the problems at hand, but also to preventive medicine and periodic health services.
  - Vaccinations.
  - Periodic screening tests: Pap smear, stool guaiacs, cholesterol, etc.
  - Counseling: Exercise, diet, disease prevention.
- Much outpatient contact occurs on the telephone; these conversations should be recorded in the chart.
- Plans for communicating test results should be documented.
- There should be a plan for follow-up.

Sample Outpatient Note

Your patient, a 52-year-old woman with hypercholesterolemia, has come for follow-up care 2 weeks after laparoscopic cholecystectomy.

December 7, 1995 Follow-Up

S: 1. Pt notes mild incisional tenderness but no other complaints. Denies fever, nausea, or abdominal pain.
2. Inquires re: estrogen replacement. Last period 2 yr previously, with severe hot flashes during first 6 mo, now moderate. She also notes mood swings but is unsure whether these are due to work-related stress or not. No dyspareunia.
3. Hypercholesterolemia: Labs 3/16/95:
Total chol, 258
HDL, 42
LDL (calc), 195
Triglycerides, 105

Pt reports working on dietary fat reduction; running 2 miles 3x/wk until surgery.

O: Temp 36.8, BP 132/84, HR 68, Wt 188 lb

HEENT: Oropharynx clear.

Neck: Supple without bruit. Thyroid normal.

Nodes: Normal.

Breasts: Normal without nodule.

Chest: Clear.

Cardiac: No JVD. PMI normal. RRR. Normal S_1, S_2 without murmur or gallop. Pulses normal.

Abdomen: Normal abdominal bowel sounds. Soft, without hepatosplenomegaly. 3 cm incision RUQ well healed without erythema, tenderness, warmth, or discharge.

Ext: No cyanosis or edema.

A: 1. Stable 2 wk after laparoscopic cholecystectomy. No evidence of perioperative complications.

2. Postmenopausal with interest in hormone replacement.
3. Hypercholesterolemia: Pt on program for dietary modification, exercise, and weight reduction.
4. Health Maintenance: Last mammogram 3 yr ago.

P: 1. Can gradually increase activity to normal.
2. Advised re: benefits and risks of hormone replacement, including potential reduction in osteoporosis, heart disease, and menopausal symptoms weighted against possible increased risk of breast and endometrial cancer. Pt will consider.
3. Reviewed calcium requirements.
4. Continue diet/exercise program.
5. Check chol, HDL, triglycerides.
6. Screening mammogram.

Pt to call in 1 wk to review results and to discuss estrogen replacement.

Follow-up 3 mo.

Bill Heberden MS3/Bigwig
HEBERDEN
BP 1234

Sample Admission Note

You have just admitted Alexander Platz from the emergency room.

August 1, 1995 9:30 PM MS Admission Note

CC: Mr. Platz is a 62-year-old man presenting because of fever and cough for 2 days.

HPI: The patient was well until 10 days ago, when he developed nasal congestion, sore throat, and low-grade fever. These seemed to improve until 2 days ago, when he noted fever to 103, cough productive of green sputum, and shortness of breath while climbing stairs.

He reports diffuse muscle aches and mild nausea but

denies shaking chills, chest pain, headache, stiff neck, or abdominal pain. No recent travel, no bird exposure, no TB exposure. He reports chronic cough productive of about a teaspoon of yellow sputum in the morning for several years but no history of lung disease, asthma, dyspnea, asbestos exposure, or hemoptysis.

PMH: MI 3 yr ago without complication or subsequent chest pain. Stress test before discharge "OK" per patient; no subsequent work-up.

Medications:	Diltiazem-CD 180 mg QD.
	Aspirin prn.
Allergies:	None known.
Smoking:	1 ppd for 40 years.
EtOH:	2 beers a day.
HIV risk factors:	None known.

Social: He works as a banana importer and is married with two children. No unusual travel.

Family History

Father:	CVA age 64.
Mother:	Alive and well.
Sister:	Lyme disease.

No cancer, heart disease, DM.

Review of Systems

General:	20 lb weight loss over 6 mo without dieting.
	No fevers, sweats, lymphadenopathy.
HEENT:	No trauma, headache, dizziness.
	No visual difficulty, pain, glaucoma, cataract.
	No auditory difficulty, pain, tinnitus.
	No discharge, breathing difficulty, sinus symptoms, epistaxis.
	No dental problems, gum bleeding, sores, change in taste.
Neck:	No voice change, difficulty swallowing, pain.
Resp:	See above.
Cardiac:	No chest pain, dyspnea, orthopnea, PND, palpitations, MI, murmur, rheumatic fever.
GI:	No abdominal pain, nausea, vomiting, liver disease, gallbladder disease, pancreatic disease, diarrhea, constipation, change in bowel habits, rectal bleeding, food intolerance.

Renal: Nocturia once nightly without hesitancy, dribbling, or retention. No kidney disease, dysuria, hematuria, UTIs.

Genital: No penile discharge, sexual difficulties, sexually transmitted disease, scrotal or testicular mass.

Back: No back pain, disk disease.

Musc. Skel: No joint pain, stiffness, swelling.

Ext: No edema, pain, phlebitis, varicosities, claudication.

Skin: No rash, growths, itching, easy bruising, change in moles, change in skin texture.

Neuro: No headache, dizziness, seizure, motor or sensory disturbance, bowel or bladder dysfunction.

Physical Examination

Mildly ill-appearing, no apparent distress

Temp 39.2, BP 150/94, HR 104, RR 28

HEENT: Conjunctivae clear without infection or discharge.

Fundi: Mild arteriolar narrowing without AV nicking or exudates.

TM nl.

Oropharynx mildly injected without exudate.

Neck: Supple without bruit; thyroid normal.

Nodes: Normal.

Chest: Coarse breath sounds in the right lower field with E to A changes.

No dullness.

Cardiac: No JVD. PMI normal. Regular rate and rhythm. Normal S_1 and S_2 without murmur or gallop. Pulses normal.

Abdomen: Normal abdominal bowel sounds. Soft, nontender, without hepatosplenomegaly.

GU: Normal penis and testes.

Rectal: Normal tone without mass. Prostate mildly enlarged without nodule. Stool brown, guaiac positive.

Skin: Normal.

Back: Normal.

Ext: Normal.

Neuro: Alert, oriented × 3. HIF normal. CN normal. Motor 5/5. Sensory intact to pin, vibration, and proprioception. DTR 2/4. Plantar reflexes downgoing.

Labs

```
         15.2
16.8>───────────<270K (84 p, 6 b, 10 l)
          45

  140 | 105 | 12
  ────┼─────┼────< 96
  3.9 |  27 | .9
```

UA: Normal.
CXR: RLL infiltrate.
Sputum Gram's Stain: Numerous polys, numerous Gram-positive cocci in clusters.

Summary: In summary, Mr. Platz is a 62-year-old man with a history of MI and smoking who presents with fever and cough for 2 days. Review of systems is remarkable for involuntary 20-lb weight loss and for mild nocturia. The exam is notable for temperature 39.2, HR 104, RR 28, moderate respiratory distress, and rhonchi with egophony in the right lower field. Guaiac-positive stool and mild prostatic enlargement are also noted. Labs are notable for WBC 16.8 with left shift. Chest x-ray demonstrates RLL infiltrate, and sputum Gram's stain reveals Gram-positive cocci in clusters.

Impression

1. ***Fever, Cough:*** Together with lung exam and RLL infiltrate, these imply right lower lobe pneumonia. Most likely organism is *S. aureus*, given Gram's stain and occurrence after an apparent URI. Pneumococcus and anaerobes are also possible. Smoking history raises the possibility of *H. influenzae* or Gram-negative rods; possibility of Legionella is raised by GI symptoms.
2. ***Guaiac-Positive Stool:*** Although gastritis and peptic ulcer disease are possible, given aspirin use, GI malignancy must be ruled out, especially considering weight loss. Other considerations include colonic polyps, diverticulosis, and AV malformations. No history of iron supplement to suggest false-positive test.
3. ***20-lb Weight Loss:*** DDx includes:

Malignancy: Lung and colon are suggested by pneumonia and guaiac-positive stool. Prostate is possible but not suggested by exam.

Chronic Infection: TB, HIV.

Collagen vascular disease doubtful.

Hyperthyroidism: Possible, but no positive evidence.

Depression.

4. ***Smoking:*** Evidence of chronic bronchitis.
5. ***BP:*** Increased at present. Diltiazem is being given at intermediate dose and could be increased if BP remains increased; however, current BP could be transiently elevated due to pt's acute illness.
6. ***H/O MI:*** Asymptomatic on diltiazem.
7. ***Prostate:*** Mild BPH by history and exam. No evidence of malignancy by exam.

Plan

1. Empiric antibiotic coverage with ampicillin-sulbactam 3 g IVSS q 6 hr.
2. If worse, add erythromycin 1 g IVSS q 6 hr to cover Legionella.
3. O_2 5 L by nasal cannula.
4. Cultures of sputum and blood.
5. PPD and controls.
6. ABG.
7. Sputum cytology × 3.
8. Repeat CXR after resolution of pneumonia to evaluate possibility of mass; consider chest CT.
9. Consider HIV testing.
10. Continue diltiazem.
    If sustained high BP, increase to CD 240 mg QD.
11. Colonoscopy when stable.
12. D/C aspirin.
13. PSA.
14. Counseling re: D/C smoking.
15. Pneumococcal vaccine when acute illness has resolved.
16. Outpatient stress-thallium test.

Bill Helvender MS3
HEBERDEN
Bp 1234

Sample Progress Notes

Sample Progress Note #1

Mr. Platz has been in the hospital for 3 days.

August 4, 1995 4 PM MS Progress Note

S: Feels well. Reports decreased cough. Walked in hall today with mild dyspnea. Reports no bowel movement since admission.

O: Tmax 37.4, BP 130–148/80–86, HR 72–88, RR 18

Oropharynx: Clear.

Chest: Coarse BS right lower field with E → A changes.

Cardiac: No JVD. RRR. nl S_1 S_2without murmur.

Abd: NABS. Mild lower abdominal distention, nontender, without HSM.

Ext: No C/E.

Labs: Sputum Cx: *S aureus*, sensitive to nafcillin, cefazolin, ampicillin-sulbactam, erythromycin; resistant to PCN, ampicillin.

13.8

10.4 >——< 182 K (90 p, 1 b)

45

134	105	10	< 86
3.2	27	.8	

PSA 1.2 mg/ml

PPD: 4-mm erythema without induration.

A:
1. RLL pneumonia. Improving. Patient now afebrile with decreasing WBC. Dyspnea improved.
2. GI. Constipation as noted. May be due to decreased activity and changed diet in hospital, although presence of guaiac-positive stool could indicate constricting colonic lesion.
3. Hypokalemia—mild.
4. Weight loss. No new findings to date; PPD negative.
5. Prostate. PSA normal, arguing against prostate cancer. Overall picture consistent with BPH.

P: 1. Change ampicillin-sulbactam to cefazolin 2 g IVSS q 6 hr.
2. MOM 30 mL PO q 12 hr; if no results, senna laxative.
3. K^+ replacement with potassium chloride 20 mEq PO BID for 3 days.
4. Consider colonoscopy; will discuss with Dr. Chiefrez.

Sample Progress Note #2

Ms. Rumplemeyer is a 59-year-old woman who was admitted 2 days ago because of hematuria. She was treated initially with a Foley catheter and is undergoing a urologic evaluation. She was also found to have an elevated alkaline phosphatase. Today, she says that she feels short of breath when she walks; this has not occurred before.

Bill Heberden MS3
HEBERDEN
BP 1234

August 31, 1995 9 AM MS Progress Note

S: Patient reports new dyspnea with walking. Denies chest pain, cough, orthopnea, or wheezing.

O: Tmax 38.2 (tympanic), BP 142/88, HR 128 irregular, RR 22

Oropharynx: Clear.

Chest: Dry crackles 1/4 on right, base only on left.

Cardiac: JVP 7 cm. Rhythm irregularly irregular. Normal S_1, S_2 with S_3, no murmur.

Abd: NABS. Soft, nontender, without HSM.

Ext: No C/E. Homans' sign negative; no cord.

EKG: AFib at 112 bpm. Axis +36°. Flattened T waves V_5–V_6 (these unchanged).

Labs

ABG (RA) 7.48/32/76/92% sat,
A-a gradient = 36
CBC pending
gamma-GTP 25

A:

1. New atrial fibrillation with rapid ventricular response. Leading potential causes include myocardial ischemia and pulmonary embolism. Fluid overload leading to increased LA pressure is possible, while less likely causes include anemia leading to increased sympathetic drive, valvular disease, and hyperthyroidism. Pt tolerating AFib fairly well despite signs of pulmonary vascular congestion.
2. New rales with increased A-a gradient and tachypnea. Probably due to AFib with decreased atrial function and increased LA pressure; PE remains possible.
3. *Hematuria:* Stable for present. Cytology sent × 2; results still pending.
4. Increased alk phos with normal G-GTP indicates bone source, raising possibility of metastatic renal or bladder Ca. Other possibilities include other metastasis (e.g., breast) or Paget's disease.

P:

1. CXR stat.
2. Digoxin 0.5 mg IVP given for rate control. Additional digoxin 0.25 mg IVP q 6 hr to maintain ventricular rate <100.
3. Change fluids to KVO.
4. Furosemide 20 mg IVP now.
5. NTP 1″ to chest wall q 4 hr.
6. O_2 4L NC.
7. V/Q scan today.
8. Will hold empiric heparinization pending results of V/Q.
9. Echocardiogram.
10. ROMI protocol with bed rest, serial cardiac enzymes, and EKGs.

11. If any signs of clinical deterioration occur → consult Telemetry Unit.
12. TFTs.
13. When stable → consider cystoscopy and IVP.
14. Probable bone scan when stable.

Discussed with Drs. Preussenkopf and Piddlekwatch.

Bill Heberden MS3 / [illegible]
HEBERDEN
BP 1234

Six hours later, you have treated the patient and observed her response. Additional data are in. It is important to record the new findings.

August 31, 1995 3 PM MS Addendum

Patient now breathing more comfortably after digoxin 0.75 mg IVP, furosemide 20 mg IVP, NTP 1″ q 4 hr.

BP 132/82, HR 88 irregular

Chest:	Few bibasilar rales
Cardiac:	JVP 5 cm. Irreg irreg, Normal S_1, S_2 without S_3.
CXR:	Mild pulm vascular congestion.
V/Q:	Matched subsegmental defect R base. Low probability for PE.
CPK #1:	34.
Repeat EKG:	AFib at 84. No ischemic changes.
CBC:	WBC 6.7, Hgb 14.1, plt 223 K.
TFTs:	Pending.

Impression: Clinically stable after above Rx for new AFib. PE unlikely.

Plan

1. Digoxin 0.25 mg PO QD.
2. Continue ROMI protocol.
3. Heparin relatively contraindicated given recent hematuria.
4. If persistent AFib, consider cardioversion with quinidine or procainamide.
5. Urologic plans as above.

Bill Heberden MS3
HEBERDEN
BP 1234

CHAPTER 5

Oral Presentations

General Principles

1. The oral presentation is an indispensable means of transmitting clinical information. The way this information is transmitted, and the level of completeness, varies according to the clinical setting.
   - Formal case presentation
   - Morning Rounds with house staff
   - Work Rounds with house staff
   - Sign-Out Rounds with house staff
2. Distinguish two separate purposes in case presentation: to transmit crucial information to another member of the health-care team, and to show someone that you know how to gather and to report clinical data. This latter function is best left for a didactic session, such as meeting with your clerkship tutor.
3. Remember that others are listening to you. Their ability to care for your patient will depend in great measure on the accuracy of the data you provide them. Furthermore, they will be able to organize the information regarding your patient best if it is presented in a way that allows them to organize it in their own minds. Finding the right balance of completeness and concision is difficult; you might consider practicing before a colleague or using a tape recorder before formally presenting cases.

Formal Case Presentation

The setting for a formal case presentation is a formal didactic session, such as the tutorial seminar in the third-year clerkship, or Grand Rounds. Its purpose is to transmit clinical information and to demonstrate that you have obtained a complete medical history, performed a complete physical examination, and analyzed the differential diagnosis, test planning, diagnosis, and treatment. Its duration should be 5 to 10 minutes, and the style is somewhat formal.

Example. Alexander Platz and His Pneumonia

Mr. Platz is a 62-year-old man presenting because of fever and cough for 2 days. He was well until 10 days ago, when he developed nasal congestion, sore throat and low-grade fever. These seemed to improve until 2 days ago, when he noted fever to 103, cough productive of green sputum, and shortness of breath while climbing stairs.

He reports diffuse muscle aches and mild nausea but denies shaking chills, chest pain, headache, stiff neck, or abdominal pain. There is no recent travel, no bird exposure, and no TB exposure. He reports chronic cough productive of about a teaspoon of yellow sputum in the morning for several years but no history of lung disease, asthma, dyspnea, asbestos exposure, or hemoptysis.

The Past Medical History is significant for an MI 3 yr ago without complication or subsequent chest pain. Medications include Diltiazem-CD 180 mg QD and aspirin prn. There are no known drug allergies. He has smoked 1 ppd for 40 years and drinks two beers a day. There are no known HIV risk factors.

He works as a banana importer and is married with two children. There is no history of unusual travel. Family History is notable for a stroke in his father and Lyme disease in his sister.

The Review of Systems is notable for a 20-lb weight loss over 6 mo without dieting. There are no fevers, sweats, lymphadenopathy.

He denies head trauma, headache, or dizziness.

He denies visual difficulty, pain, glaucoma, or cataract.

There is no auditory difficulty, pain, or tinnitus.

There is no nasal discharge, breathing difficulty, sinus symptoms, or epistaxis.

There are no dental problems, gum bleeding, sores, or change in taste.

He denies voice change, difficulty swallowing, or neck pain.

He denies chest pain, dyspnea, orthopnea, PND, palpitations, murmur, or rheumatic fever.

There is no abdominal pain, nausea, vomiting, liver disease, gallbladder disease, pancreatic disease, diarrhea, constipation, change in bowel habits, rectal bleeding, or food intolerance.

He denies kidney disease, dysuria, hematuria, nocturia, or urinary tract infections.

He reports nocturia once nightly but denies hesitancy, dribbling, penile discharge, sexual difficulties, sexually transmitted disease, or scrotal or testicular mass.

There is no back pain or disk disease.

He denies joint pain, stiffness, or swelling.

He denies edema, pain, phlebitis, varicosities, or claudication.

He denies rash, skin growths, itching, easy bruising, change in moles, or change in skin texture.

He denies headache, dizziness, seizure, motor or sensory disturbance, or bowel or bladder dysfunction.

On exam, the patient was mildly ill-appearing, in moderate respiratory distress. Temperature was 39.7 tympanic with BP 150/94, HR 104, RR 28.

The head was normal. The extraocular structures

were intact. The conjunctivae were mildly injected without discharge. The sclera were clear. Optic disks were flat, and the fundi had mild arteriolar narrowing but no AV nicking, exudates, or hemorrhages.

The pinnae, auditory canals, and tympanic membranes were normal. The external nasal structures and nares were normal. The oropharynx demonstrated good dentition with no lesions of the buccal mucosa, gums, or pharynx.

The neck was supple without bruit. The thyroid was normal.

There were no palpable lymph nodes.

Examination of the chest revealed coarse crackles in the right lower field with E to A changes but no dullness.

There was no JVD. The carotid upstrokes were normal. The apical impulse was palpable in the left fifth intercostal space, midclavicular line. S_1 and S_2 were normal. There was no murmur, gallop, or rub. Pulses were normal.

The abdomen had normal active bowel sounds and was soft and nontender. The liver was 12 cm by percussion and was smooth, firm, and nontender. The spleen was not palpable. There were no masses and no hernia.

The penis and testes were normal.

The rectal exam showed normal tone without mass. The prostate was mildly enlarged but had no nodule or asymmetry. The stool was brown and *guaiac positive* for occult blood.

The back was symmetric and nontender. The skin had no abnormal findings. The extremities had no cyanosis, clubbing, or edema.

On neurologic exam, the patient was alert and oriented × 3. Higher intellectual function was normal. Cranial nerves II–XII were normal. Strength and tone were normal. Sensation was intact to pin, temperature, vibration, and proprioception. Rapid alternating motion was normal. The gait was normal. Deep tendon reflexes were 2/4 throughout. The plantar reflexes were downgoing.

Lab studies were notable for WBC 16.8 with 84% polys, 6% bands, and 10% lymphs. Chest x-ray demonstrates right lower lobe infiltrate. Sputum Gram's stain revealed numerous polys and numerous Gram-positive cocci in clusters.

In summary, Mr. Platz is a 62-year-old man with a history of MI and smoking who presents with fever and cough for 2 days. Review of Systems is remarkable for involuntary 20-lb weight loss, for chronic productive cough, and for mild nocturia. The exam is notable for temperature 39.7, HR 104, RR 28, moderate respiratory distress, and rhonchi with egophony in the right lower field. Guaiac-positive stool and mild prostatic enlargement are also noted. Labs are notable for WBC 16.8 with left shift. Chest x-ray demonstrates RLL infiltrate, and sputum Gram's stain reveals Gram-positive cocci in clusters.

Presentation on Morning Rounds

1. The setting for presentation on Morning Rounds is related to work. The house staff, students, and teaching faculty are gathered to review admissions from the previous day. The purpose of a Morning Rounds presentation is to transmit clinical information. By the end of your presentation, the other members of the team should know everything about the patient that might be pertinent to his or her care. Its duration is ≤5 minutes and the style is concise.
2. The presentation is formatted to meet these ends. The Chief Complaint, History of the Present Ill-

ness, and Past Medical History are reported as in the formal case presentation, stressing concision. The Social History, Family History, and Review of Systems are reduced to noteworthy findings only. The Physical Exam describes the neck, lymph nodes, respiratory, cardiac, abdomen, rectal, and extremities exams in full. Other organ systems are described only if abnormal. Labs and Summary are described as in the formal exam.

Example. Alexander Platz Again

Mr. Platz is a 62-year-old man presenting because of fever and cough for 2 days. He was well until 10 days ago, when he developed nasal congestion, sore throat, and low-grade fever. These seemed to improve until 2 days ago, when he noted fever to 103, cough productive of green sputum, and shortness of breath while climbing stairs.

He reports diffuse muscle aches and mild nausea but denies shaking chills, chest pain, headache, stiff neck, or abdominal pain. There is no recent travel, no bird exposure, and no TB exposure. He reports chronic cough productive of about a teaspoon of yellow sputum in the morning for several years but no history of lung disease, asthma, dyspnea, asbestos exposure, or hemoptysis.

The Past Medical History is significant for an MI 3 yr ago without complication or subsequent chest pain. Medications include Diltiazem-CD 180 mg QD and aspirin prn. There are no known drug allergies. He has smoked 1 ppd for 40 years and drinks two beers a day. There are no known HIV risk factors.

He works as a banana importer and is married with two children. There is no history of unusual travel. Family History is notable for a stroke in his father.

The Review of Systems is notable for a 20-lb weight

loss over 6 mo without dieting. There are no fevers, sweats, or lymphadenopathy.

He denies chest pain, dyspnea, orthopnea, PND, palpitations, murmur, or rheumatic fever.

There is no abdominal pain, nausea, vomiting, liver disease, gallbladder disease, pancreatic disease, diarrhea, constipation, change in bowel habits, rectal bleeding, or food intolerance.

He denies kidney disease, dysuria, hematuria, nocturia, or urinary tract infections.

He reports nocturia once nightly but denies hesitancy, dribbling, penile discharge, sexual difficulties, sexually transmitted disease, or scrotal or testicular mass.

On exam, the patient was mildly ill-appearing, in moderate respiratory distress. Temperature was 39.7 tympanic with BP $^{150}/_{94}$. HR 104, RR 28.

The head was normal. The eyes were normal except for mild arteriolar narrowing. The ears, nose, and mouth were normal.

The neck was supple without bruit. The thyroid was were normal.

There were no palpable lymph nodes.

The chest had coarse crackles in the right lower field with E to A changes but no dullness.

There was no JVD. The carotid upstrokes were normal. The apical impulse was palpable in the left fifth intercostal space, midclavicular line. S_1 and S_2 were normal. There was no murmur, gallop, or rub. Pulses were normal.

The abdomen had normal active bowel sounds and was soft and nontender. The liver was 12 cm by percussion and was smooth, firm, and nontender. The spleen was not palpable. There were no masses and no hernia.

The penis and testes were normal.

The rectal exam showed normal tone without mass.

The prostate was mildly enlarged but had no nodule or asymmetry. The stool was brown and *guaiac positive* for occult blood.

The back, skin, and extremities were normal.

On neurologic exam, the patient was alert and oriented × 3. Higher intellectual function was normal. Cranial nerves II–XII were normal. Strength and tone were normal. Sensation was intact to pin, temperature, vibration, and proprioception. Rapid alternating motion was normal. The gait was normal. Deep tendon reflexes were 2/4 throughout. The plantar reflexes were downgoing.

Lab studies were notable for WBC 16.8 and 84% polys, 6% bands, and 10% lymphs. Chest x-ray demonstrates right lower lobe infiltrate. Sputum Gram's stain revealed numerous polys and numerous Gram-positive cocci in clusters.

In summary, Mr. Platz is a 62-year-old man with a history of MI and smoking who presents with fever and cough for 2 days. Review of Systems is remarkable for involuntary 20-lb weight loss, for chronic productive cough, and for mild nocturia. The exam is notable for temperature 39.7, HR 104, RR 28, moderate respiratory distress, and rhonchi with egophony in the right lower field. Guaiac-positive stool and mild prostatic enlargement are also noted. Labs are notable for WBC 16.8 with left shift. Chest x-ray demonstrates RLL infiltrate, and sputum Gram's stain reveals Gram positive cocci in clusters.

Other Presentations

Other presentation styles are used depending on the need for concision. To tell a new member of the medical team about Mr. Platz, you might use the following version of his story:

Example

> Mr. Platz is a 62-year-old man admitted because of fever, cough, and dyspnea for 2 days. PMH notable for uncomplicated MI 2 yr ago and for chronic cough. Exam notable for temp 39.7, moderate respiratory distress, and rhonchi with egophony in the right lower field. Labs are notable for WBC 16.8 with left shift. Chest x-ray demonstrates RLL infiltrate, and sputum Gram's stain reveals Gram-positive cocci in clusters. Other issues include 20-lb weight loss and guaiac-positive stool. Treatment includes ampicillin-sulbactam IV; if worse, erythromycin IV will be added. Other plans include colonoscopy when stable.

At the end of the day, to tell the covering physician (or student) what they need to know about Mr. Platz, the following version would be best:

Example

> Mr. Smith is a 62-year-old man admitted with apparent RLL pneumonia, being treated with ampicillin-sulbactam IV. Other issues include h/o MI, 20-lb weight loss, and guaiac-positive stool. If he gets worse, add erythromycin IV.

CHAPTER 6

Writing Orders

General Principles

1. Orders are a doctor's instructions given to another health-care provider. The provider may be a nurse, a nurse's assistant, a pharmacist, a radiology technician—in fact, anyone within the medical system.
2. Calling a medical instruction an *order* makes it sound like a military order from an officer to a subordinate. In fact, a medical order has an intermediate level of authority: less than a command, but more than a request. The person receiving the order is expected to carry it out, *if* there is no medical contraindication. A provider must not do something that he or she feels is unsafe. For example, if you order a medication to which a patient is allergic, the nurse should not give the medication without discussing the allergy with you. If insulin has been ordered but the patient is found to have a low blood glucose already, the insulin should not be given without consulting the ordering physician.
3. An order must be clear and unambiguous. The person reading an order should be able to tell exactly what is to be done, and there should be only one possible interpretation.
4. It never hurts to say "*Please*."

How to Write an Order

1. *Make it legible.* An order must be legible. Major mistakes, some fatal, have been made when an order was read incorrectly because of unclear handwriting. If your script is unclear, print.
2. Know where to write your orders. This could be:
   - *The order book.* Usually this is a loose-leaf book kept at the nursing station.
   - *Order sheets.* A set of special sheets are kept either in the patient's chart or at the patient's bedside.
   - *A computer.* Many medical centers have on-line ordering. The principles are identical to written orders.
3. *Date and time all orders.*
4. *Write it.* All orders must be written. By design, the order should be written before action is taken. Verbal or telephone orders are sometimes given either for emergencies, when time is of the essence, or for the sake of convenience on minor issues. Verbal orders must all be written at some point, so it is a good habit simply to write all orders.

   Nurses will usually not act on verbal orders from medical students.
5. *Sign it.* As a medical student, you should:
   - Sign your name.
   - Follow your signature with an indication of your function on the medical team. A third-year student typically writes, MS 3 (the *MS* stands for *Medical Student*). At some medical schools, the student writes the school's initials or other tag instead of *MS*. Interns and residents simply write *MD*.
   - Print your name underneath the signature.
   - If you carry a beeper, write the beeper number under or beside your name. This allows someone to contact you if there is any question.
6. All orders must be signed by a physician. You should ensure that your orders have been *counter-*

signed by a physician, usually your intern or resident.

7. *Flag the order.* Each hospital has a system for indicating that an order has been written: writing the patient's name on the front of the order book, or raising a plastic tag on the chart.

   If the order needs prompt action, tell the nurse in person.
8. *Confirm* that the order has been properly executed. Hospitals keep a written record, often called a *Medex*, of every medication that has been given to a patient. You should check this record daily. By checking the Medex, you:
   - Know exactly what your patient is receiving.
   - Ensure that a medication you ordered is being properly administered.
   - Avoid surprises. Examples of unpleasant surprises include:
     - The patient refused to take the medicine.
     - The patient was unable to take the medicine.
     - The nurse decided not to give the medicine. For example, an antihypertensive medication was not given because the blood pressure was too low.
     - Someone else ordered a medicine for your patient that you didn't know about.
     - A medication was started a week ago and you forgot to stop it.

Ordering Medications

1. A proper order for a medication includes:
   - Name of the medicine
   - Dose
   - How given (orally, intravenously, etc.)
   - How often
   - How long
   - Special instructions, if needed

2. Medicines can be called by their generic or trade names. In general, the generic name is preferred. However, some medications are so commonly indicated by their trade names that using their generic names is stilted and pedantic. Local usage dictates.
3. **Dose.** The proper dose of a medication may depend on a number of variables, including:
   - **Patient Age.** In general, older patients require lower doses. For children, doses are virtually always adjusted for age, weight, or both.
   - **Body Weight.** In general, heavier patients require higher doses. Some medicines are dosed specifically by the patient's actual weight. Examples include:
     - Aminoglycoside antibiotics, such as gentamicin
     - Cardiovascular pressor agents, such as dopamine
     - Cancer chemotherapeutic agents, such as 5-fluorouracil
     - Certain antiviral agents, such as didanosine (ddI)
     - Most pediatric medications, especially in infants

     Some medications (mostly cancer chemotherapeutic agents) are dosed according to body surface area, which is estimated from body weight and height.
   - **Condition Being Treated.** More serious conditions often require higher doses.
   - **Prior Medication Use.** In general, one starts at low doses and then increases. This reduces the chance of side effects.
   - **Concurrent Medications.** A medication may interact with another, by affecting absorption, binding to carrier proteins, drug metabolism, receptor sites, or other features of drug action. While any medication might have an interaction with another, certain medications have a high pro-

pensity for drug interactions. These include: antiepileptics (especially barbiturates), warfarin, cimetidine, tricyclic antidepressants, monoamine oxidase inhibitors, phenothiazines, and oral contraceptives.

- **Kidney Function.** *Many* drugs are excreted in the urine and should be given in reduced doses when kidney function is impaired. This applies in particular to antibiotics. Drug references always indicate when doses should be reduced according to kidney function. As a rule of thumb, check dosing adjustments whenever the estimated creatinine clearance is below 50 mL/hr.

Kidney function can be approximated by a formula:

Creatinine clearance (mL/hr) =

$$(140 - \text{age})/\text{creatinine} \times \text{body weight (kg)}/70$$

The result is multiplied by 0.8 for women.

Always consider whether a patient's kidney function might be less than is immediately apparent. An 80-year-old woman who weighs 100 lb (45 kg) and has a serum creatinine of 1.5 has an estimated creatinine clearance of:

$$(140 - 80)/1.5 \times 45/70 \times 0.8 = 20.5 \text{ mL/hr}$$

Her medication doses need to be reduced appropriately This is often accomplished by increasing the dosing interval (i.e., by giving the drug less frequently). All drug references should describe dosing adjustment for renal and hepatic function.

An excellent reference for dosing medications in patients with renal disease is published by the American College of Physicians: Bennett, WM, et al: *Drug Prescribing in Renal Failure: Dosing Guidelines for Adults,* ed 3. Philadelphia, American College of Physicians, 1994.

- **Liver Function.** Some medications that are processed by the liver should be given in reduced doses when liver function is impaired. Notable examples include benzodiazepines, antiepileptics, opioids, warfarin, and certain antibiotics. Again, look up the possible effect of hepatic insufficiency whenever liver function might be impaired, as in hepatitis, jaundice of any cause, or cirrhosis.
- **Tolerance.** A patient who has been taking regular doses of benzodiazepines, opioids, barbiturates, or other agents will require higher doses of these agents to have a pharmacologic effect than someone who has never taken the medication.
- **Blood Levels.** For some medications, the drug level (or some other measurement of drug activity) is measured and the dose is adjusted to achieve a target level. Examples include antiepileptics, certain tricyclic antidepressants, theophylline, digoxin, quinidine, and procainamide.
- **Other Target Effects.** Dosages of the anticoagulants warfarin and heparin are determined by measuring clotting tests: the prothrombin time (PT) for the former, and the partial thromboplastin time (PTT) for the latter. Hydroxyurea decreases platelet production and is given in whatever dose brings the platelet count to a desired range. Insulin is adjusted to achieve normal glucose levels. Nitroprusside, which is given by continuous infusion, may be adjusted minute-to-minute to achieve a target blood pressure.

4. **How the Medication Is to Be Given.** Options include:
   - **Oral (PO).** The medication is swallowed.
   - **Intravenous (IV).** The medication is injected into a vein. Variants include:
     - IV push (IVP). The medication is given in a small volume (0.1 to 100 mL) that is injected rapidly.

   - IV Soluset® (IVSS). The medication is given in a volume of 50 to 500 mL that is infused over 10 to 60 minutes. Most parenteral antibiotics are given this way.
   - IV infusion. The medication is given by pump at a constant, specified rate. Medications given by IV infusion include heparin, aminophylline, cardiovascular pressors, and cancer chemotherapeutic agents.
- **Intramuscular (IM)**. The traditional "shot."
- **Subcutaneous (SC or SQ)**. The medicine is injected under the skin.
- **Sublingual (SL)**. The medication is placed under the tongue and allowed to dissolve. Nitroglycerin is commonly given this way.
- **Rectal (PR)**. A suppository is placed in the rectum and allowed to dissolve.
- **Cutaneous**. An ointment or creme is applied to the skin.
- **Miscellaneous** routes include the eye, ear, nose, and vagina. One nitroglycerin preparation is sprayed on the inside of the cheek.

5. **How Often the Medication Is to Be Given**. The frequency of dosing is based on the absorption and elimination of the drug. Options include:
   - Daily (QD).
   - More than once daily: twice (BID), three times (TID), four times (QID)
   - Less than once daily: every other day (QOD), once weekly, etc.
   - At specified hourly intervals: every *n* hours (usually a factor of 24). This is written as q6hr, q24hr, etc.
   - *Caution:* be careful to distinguish QD (daily) from QID (4 times daily)

   What is the difference between *q8hr* and *TID*? A medication ordered *q8hr* will be usually be given at 8 AM, 4 PM, and midnight. A medication ordered

TID will be given at breakfast, supper, and bedtime, or some similar arrangement, at the convenience of the patient and the nurse. Specifying the interval by *q8hr* is important when high degrees of precision are necessary, as in certain cardiovascular medications. Otherwise, *TID* is more convenient.

Dosing *intervals* must often be adjusted in the same way as doses. In renal or hepatic insufficiency, a drug may be given less frequently.

6. **Duration.** Antibiotics are usually given for a specified period (e.g., 10 days), which should be specified. Other medications are typically given indefinitely, or "until further notice."
7. *Special instructions* you might give regarding the order:
   - A *"Hold" order* indicates that a medicine should not be given under some circumstances. For instance, a sedative should not be given if the patient is already lethargic.
   - *PRN* means that the medication is given only as someone chooses. Either the patient or the nurse may initiate the transaction; the patient may request the medication or the nurse may offer it. *PRN orders should always specify the circumstances under which the medication is to be used. If you write, "Acetaminophen 650 mg PO q 4 hr prn," you may find that the nurse gives the medicine every time the patient has a fever, while you intended it to be used for headache.*
   - *STAT* (from Latin *statim*, "immediately") means that the order should be considered urgent. STAT should be used for medical emergencies, not for someone's convenience.
8. A word on abbreviations. Abbreviations are used universally in medicine. The view expressed in some pharmacology texts, that abbreviations are dangerously prone to error and should therefore be

avoided, is impracticable. You should, however, restrict your use to the commonly used abbreviations. These are listed in Appendix 1.

Examples

Ceftriaxone 1 g IVSS q 24 hr × 10 days

This means that the antibiotic ceftriaxone should be given as 1 g by intravenous infusion every 24 hours for 10 days.

Specifying a definite duration of treatment is a good idea for most antibiotics; otherwise, someone may forget to stop the drug.

Metoprolol 25 mg PO q 12 hr please
Hold for BP <100/50, HR <50

Metoprolol is a beta blocker that reduces blood pressure and heart rate. You indicate that it should not be given if the BP or HR are already below a specified threshold.

Aluminum hydroxide antacid 30 mL PO q 4 hr prn indigestion

PRN means that the medicine should be given as needed for a certain problem. In this instance, the antacid should be given if the patient develops indigestion but not otherwise.

Morphine sulfate 4 mg SC q 4 hr ATC; patient may refuse

ATC means around the clock. The plan here is to offer a patient who has severe pain a strong analgesic, allowing the patient to say no. This avoids the delay that can occur when a patient has to ask for a medicine before the nurse goes to the medication supplies, finds the medicine, and administers it.

Furosemide 40 mg IVP × 1; given

If you give a medication yourself, you should still write an order for it but indicate that the order has been executed.

Ordering Fluids

1. There are several **types of fluid** for intravenous administration.
   - **Normal Saline** (NS). Sodium chloride at a concentration of 154 mEq/L, dissolved in water. Best for short-term fluid replacement in patients who are volume depleted.
   - **Lactated Ringer's Solution.** A combination of sodium chloride and lactate. Better than NS for longer-term fluid replacement in volume-depleted patients; because some of the anion is provided as lactate, the patient receives less chloride and is less prone to develop a hyperchloremic metabolic acidosis.
   - $\frac{1}{2}$ **Normal Saline** ($\frac{1}{2}$ NS). Sodium chloride at 77 mEq/L. The best choice for patients who are euvolemic (i.e., who have an appropriate fluid status) but who are unable to take oral liquids.
   - $\frac{1}{2}$ **NS + KCl 20 mEq/L.** Potassium is often added to maintenance IV fluids, either because the patient has a low serum potassium level or in order to avoid the hypokalemia that often occurs when the only cation is sodium.
   - **D5W.** 5% dextrose in water; i.e., dextrose in water at a concentration of 5 g/L. This is used when a patient requires free water but no salt. It runs the risk of hyponatremia and is not a good choice in volume depletion. *The question often arises whether D5W should be given in diabetes. If D5W is given at 75 mL/hr for 24 hr, the patient will receive 1.8 L of fluid containing 50 g/L, or 90 g of dextrose. This translates to 450 calories of sugar, about the same amount as a candy bar. Large amounts of D5W should thus be avoided, if possible, in patients with diabetes, but not if some other issue, such as hypernatremia, requires free water.*
2. **Rate of Administration.** A healthy person requires about 0.8 to 1 mL/hr/kg body weight of water. A

patient who is unable to take fluids orally needs this volume to be administered intravenously. This requirement is increased if fluid loss is increased, as in patients with burns, fevers, diarrhea, vomiting, "third-spacing," or excessive urinary loss.

A patient who is hypovolemic, after volume loss, may require considerably more fluids. Severe hypotension might require several liters of fluid given as rapidly as possible.

Rates of infusion can be estimated by controlling the drip rate of the fluid, or specified exactly using an infusion pump. Estimating the rate is adequate for most purposes; pumps must be used when precision is required. Drugs that require a precise rate of delivery, such as aminophylline, heparin, cardiovascular pressors, or cancer chemotherapeutic agents, require infusion pumps.

KVO (keep vein open) means that intravenous fluids are dripped in as slowly as possible, in a rate adequate to keep the catheter patent. The patient generally does not require additional fluids, but only a means of receiving intravenous medications. KVO usually amounts to 5 to 20 mL/hr.

3. **Route of Administration**
   - **Peripheral Catheter.** A short (3 to 10 cm) catheter that is inserted into a vein, usually on the arm or hand, and remains for up to 3 days. Fluids must be instilled continuously to avoid clotting. Peripheral catheters are best used for continuous intravenous medications, such as heparin, or for fluid administration.
   - **Heparin Lock or Saline Lock.** A similar catheter that is connected to a short (3 to 4 cm) hub. Clotting is prevented by filling the hub periodically with a heparin or saline solution. Locks of various types are best used for intermittent intravenous medications, such as antibiotics. Because heparin has been used up to the present, these catheters are often called *hep-locks*. However, it

has recently become apparent that saline works just as well and has fewer side effects.

- **Central Catheter.** A long (10 to 30 cm) catheter that is inserted, using special techniques, into a large central vein, such as the subclavian, internal jugular, or femoral vein. These are best used for administration of medications that are especially irritating to small veins, such as some chemotherapeutic agents, or of large volumes of fluids in critically ill patients. Central catheters are also used when no peripheral veins can be cannulated.
- **Peripherally Inserted Central Catheter** (PICC line). A long (60 cm) catheter is inserted into an arm vein for long-term use. It extends into the superior vena cava.

4. Examples:
   - *NS @ 75 mL/hr via peripheral catheter*
   - *D5W + KCl 40 mEq/L at 30 mL/hr via peripheral catheter; infusion pump please*
   - *Lactated Ringer's @ 500 mL over 1 hr via left subclavian catheter*

Ordering Oxygen

1. Oxygen can be given by face mask, nasal cannulae, facial tent, tracheostomy collar, or mechanical ventilator.
2. The immediate source of oxygen is either an oxygen tank or a pipe system built into the wall. The gas flowing from these devices is 100% oxygen.
3. Lesser amounts of oxygen are provided by mixing the 100% oxygen from the supply with room air, which contains on average 21% oxygen. The mixing devices on all instruments except mechanical ventilators are only approximate.
4. A *face mask* is used when substantial oxygen sup-

plementation is required. It is usually hot, tight, and uncomfortable. An adapter at the base of the mask controls how much room air is allowed to mix with the 100% oxygen that flows from the tank or wall. The order specifies the percentage of oxygen desired, indicated in increments of 10.

Example: Oxygen by 50% face mask

When 100% oxygen is required, a *nonrebreather mask* is ordered to ensure that the patient only inhales the 100% oxygen delivered from the system. This is even more uncomfortable than a regular face mask.

5. *Nasal cannulae* are little prongs that are inserted into the nostril. They are best used when modest oxygen augmentation is required. They are less precise than face masks but more comfortable. A valve at the oxygen supply adjusts the rate of flow of 100% oxygen from the tank; the remainder of the patient's inhaled gas is room air. The order specifies the rate of flow.

Example: Oxygen 2 L/min by nasal cannulae

The maximum rate of flow is 5 to 6 L/min. Note that the actual amount of oxygen the patient inhales will depend on how much he or she breathes through the nose (vs. mouth), and what the total tidal volume is. The greater the tidal volume, the greater the proportion of room air. An approximate conversion between nasal cannula flow and % oxygen delivery is as follows:

Nasal Flow (L/min)	Oxygen Delivery (%)
2	24–28
3	28–32
4	32–36
5	about 35

6. A *facial tent*, which looks like a large basin placed below the chin, is used when facial trauma or surgery would interfere with masks or cannulae.
7. A *tracheostomy* is an incision made in the trachea, below the vocal cords, for purposes of breathing and/or airway suctioning. A short L-shaped plastic tube is inserted into the incision. Air is supplied to the tracheostomy either by applying a loosely fitting collar or by attaching it to a mechanical ventilator. The tracheostomy collar can provide oxygen-enhanced air, while the ventilator can also ventilate the patient.
8. *Mechanical ventilators* are used either when the patient is unable to breath unassisted, or when very high levels of oxygen supplementation are required. Mechanical ventilators require that a tube, called an *endotracheal tube*, be placed directly into the trachea via the mouth, nose, or tracheostomy.
9. Oxygen levels in the blood can be measured in two ways.
   - **Arterial Blood Gas.** A sample of arterial blood is analyzed for pH, partial pressure of oxygen (Po_2), partial pressure of carbon dioxide (Pco_2), and % oxygen saturation (Sao_2).
   - **Pulse Oximeter.** An infrared device is placed on the patient's fingertip and measures Sao_2.

   The patient should receive enough oxygen to ensure a $Po_2 \geq 90$ mm Hg or $Sao_2 \geq 90\%$.
10. Caution is warranted in prescribing oxygen therapy. Oxygen is toxic to the eyes and the lungs when it is given in high amounts (>40% to 50%) for prolonged periods (more than 2 to 3 days). Always try to avoid this exposure if the patient's condition allows. In addition, oxygen supplementation may reduce ventilatory drive in patients with chronic obstructive pulmonary disease (COPD). A patient with COPD who is given too much oxygen may simply stop breathing.

Other Orders

The physician must specifically order virtually every aspect of medical care.

1. *Treatments*, such as blood products or wound dressings

   Examples

   - Transfuse PRBC × 2 over 4 hr please
   - Povidone wet-to-dry dressing to left foot TID

2. Tests

   Examples

   - AM labs: CBC, glucose
   - CXR portable STAT
   - Please schedule abdominal sonogram

3. **Diet.** The physician must specify what kind of food the patient is to have. Most patients can have whatever is being offered, usually a "standard" American meal consisting of meat or fish, potato or rice, bread, and a vegetable. Many patients should have a special diet, either for medical, personal, or religious reasons; examples are given in the Table.

Condition	Diet	Rationale
Diabetes	1800 cal (or 2000, or 2400), no concentrated sweets	Restrict glucose and total calories.
Coronary artery disease	Low cholesterol	Reduce atherogenesis.
Congestive heart failure	2–3 g sodium	Salt restriction.
Renal insufficiency	40 g protein, 2–3 g sodium	Protein restriction slows the progression of renal disease.

(Table continued on next page)

Condition	Diet	Rationale
Hepatic insufficiency	40 g protein	Protein restriction reduces the production of ammonia.
Before surgery	NPO after midnight	An empty stomach reduces the chance of aspiration during anesthesia.
During recovery from major surgery	Clear liquids	The bowels become relatively inactive after major surgery; food is reintroduced gradually.
Poor swallowing	Aspiration I or II diet	An aspiration diet consists of sticky foods, such as mashed potatoes or yogurt, and avoids fluids or foods that require chewing. These reduce the risk of aspiration.

4. Activity

Examples

- Out of bed ad lib
- Bed rest
- Ambulate with assistance

5. Hardware

   Examples
   - Foley catheter to straight drainage please
   - Venous compression boots
   - Bedside commode

Making Sure the Order Is Right

1. You can check with another doctor, especially one who is directly supervising you. This is the most popular method, but it is not foolproof.
2. There are several important reference texts for medications.*
   - The *American Hospital Formulary Service Drug Information* can be found in many nursing stations and in (I hope) all hospital libraries. This is published annually and represents objective, unbiased information on all drugs.
   - *Drug Facts and Comparisons* is another excellent reference, comprehensive and impartial. It is revised and published annually.
   - The *Physician's Desk Reference (PDR)* can be found at most nursing stations. The *PDR* is an annual compilation of what pharmaceutical companies say about their products on package inserts. It is not as clear as either of the other references on such topics as mechanisms of action, side effects, and comparison with other agents. It also does not provide information regarding nonprescription drugs and intravenous solutions.
3. Pocket manuals are also widely available.* The best are:
   - The Medical Letter, *Drugs of Choice*. A concise, impartial guide to common classes of medications. Not all classes of medication are covered.

---

*Full bibliographic information is given in Appendix B.

- Sanford, JP: *Guide to Antimicrobial Therapy*. Revised annually, this inexpensive volume describes, for each infectious syndrome, the common causative microorganisms and recommended antibiotics. Drug dosing and pharmacologic properties are also described. This is the publication most frequently found in interns' pockets.
- Mandell, GL, et al: *Principles and Practice of Infectious Diseases: Antimicrobial Therapy 1993/1994*. Also quite good, and cross-referenced to the two-volume textbook in Infectious Diseases.

4. Some hospitals and ambulatory practices provide computer-based references for drug information.
5. Make sure the dose is right. Run through a mental checklist regarding dose adjustment for age, weight, kidney function, liver function, concurrent medications, and drug levels.
6. Make sure there are no drug interactions or contraindications. This can be done by consulting any of the references mentioned above. In addition, several readily available references address the issue of interactions directly.
   - *The Medical Letter Handbook of Adverse Drug Interactions.*
   - *Drug Interactions and Side Effects Index.* Published by the PDR, with the same issues.

   Both are available on computer.

7. If you're not *absolutely* certain, look it up.

Admission Orders

1. Orders should be written for all patients shortly after admission. Admission orders set the initial rules.
2. A mnemonic will help you include all the relevant items.

   A B C Van Dimals

   A Admit to [*name of floor or service*]

[Name of attending, intern, you]
B "Because of" [i.e., diagnosis]
C Condition (stable, guarded, critical)
V Vital signs (what and how often)
A Activity
N Nursing
D Diet
I IV
M Medications
A Allergies
L Labs
S Special instructions

Example

Admit to Payson 5
Attending Dr. Auenbrugger, Resident Dr. Janeway, Med Student Bill Heberden, beeper 1234
Diagnosis: Pneumonia, diabetes mellitus
Condition: Stable
Vital signs: Temperature, BP, HR, RR TID
Activity: Out of bed ad lib
Nursing: Please check fingerstick glucose QID
Diet: 1800 kcal, ADA diet
IV: hep-lock; please flush with saline TID
Medications: Cefuroxime 1.5 g IVSS TID for 10 days
Glyburide 5 mg PO qD
Enalapril 5 mg PO qD
Acetaminophen 650 mg PO q 6 hr prn headache
Aluminum hydroxide antacid 30 mL PO q 6 hr prn indigestion
Milk of magnesia 30 mL PO q 12 hr prn constipation
Temazepam 30 mg PO qhs prn insomnia
Allergies: Sulfa → hives

AM Labs: CBC with differential
Glucose
Please call house officer for temp >38.5

Bill Heberden MS3
HEBERDEN
Bp 1234 / Janeway

3. Tips
   - **Diagnosis.** Note the main reason the patient is admitted and the major underlying conditions. Not every condition needs to be named here.
   - **Condition.** Some hospitals, and all movies, treat the condition as a crucial label that encapsulates the patient's proximity to death. Other hospitals treat the matter more routinely and consider all patients in Intensive Care as *critical* and all others as *stable*. Follow your hospital's customs.
   - **Vital Signs.** Some hospitals require that the type and frequency of vital signs be specified; others allow you to write, "Per routine." You may need to order vital signs more frequently in specific conditions, usually major acute illnesses.
   - **Activity.** Patients should be as active as their condition permits. Patients who are left in bed are susceptible to thromboses, decubitus ulcers, aspiration, orthostatic hypotension, osteoporosis, loss of muscle mass, and flexion contractures.
   - **Medications.** First order the new medications being started for whatever illness is at hand. Then review the medications that the patient had taken up to the point of admission. Chronic medications, such as those used to treat hypertension or heart disease, should usually be continued. But the decision to continue a medicine must be reviewed critically. For example, you should not continue di-

uretics or antihypertensives in a patient admitted with an acute gastrointestinal hemorrhage.

- **PRN Medications.** You should anticipate the minor discomforts and annoyances that may occur in the hospital. Due to changes in diet, activity, and environment, many patients develop difficulties with bowel movements or sleep in the hospital. By ordering medications to deal with these problems in advance, you provide for your patients' comfort—and also protect your fellow physicians from being awakened at 2 AM because someone can't sleep.
- **Allergies.** Drugs that have been reported to cause allergic reaction, and the nature of the reaction, should be listed.
- **Special Instructions.** Anything is possible. You may want to specify conditions under which the physician should be called; for example, for fever.

4. Think about deep venous thrombosis (DVT) and its prevention. A patient who is inactive should receive some form of DVT prophylaxis. Options include:
   - Heparin SC. The standard, usually given as 5000 U SC q 12 hr.
   - Low-molecular-weight heparin is a new alternative that may be preferred in some centers.
   - Venous compression boots. These are inflatable leggings that compress the legs and augment venous blood flow.
   - Early mobilization is important. If the patient can be out of bed a few times a day, order it (*OOB to chair TID*) instead of maintaining bed rest.
5. Admission orders must generally be rewritten any time a patient is transferred from one part of the hospital to another, or after surgery.

Daily Orders

1. Orders are generally written for each patient at least once daily, usually twice, and often more frequently.

An order should be written whenever a new treatment or test is planned. Groups of orders can be batched.

2. Some orders must be renewed. In New York, for example, oxygen, intravenous catheters, and blood products must be renewed daily. Narcotics must be renewed every 3 days. All other orders must be renewed every 7 days, unless a definite time limit is specified in the initial order.
3. Orders written in the afternoon usually request blood tests for the next day.

Preoperative Orders

1. **NPO After Midnight.** For most surgery, the patient takes nothing by mouth after the midnight before surgery. Medications, taken with a sip of water, are sometimes exempt.
2. For many abdominal or pelvic operations, enemas are given the night before surgery to evacuate the bowels.
3. **Prophylactic Antibiotics.** Antibiotics are given to prevent infection in certain operations. These include:
   - "Dirty surgery": when actual infection is suspected, as in surgery for abscess
   - Operations in which prior contamination is suspected, such as repair of open fractures or amputation
   - Procedures that incise nonsterile membranes, such as oral surgery, gastric or intestinal surgery, hysterectomy
   - Procedures for which infection could be catastrophic, such as joint replacement, aortic surgery, coronary artery bypass, etc.
4. **Sedatives.** These are often ordered *on call* to surgery; the nurse will administer them 30 to 60 minutes before the operation.
5. **Intravenous Fluids.** Most operations require a functioning IV line; ordering this in advance will prevent delay.

Postoperative Orders

1. After surgery, the patient is essentially readmitted to the hospital. All orders must be rewritten.
2. Patients who have had general anesthesia should be NPO until their gag reflex returns.
3. Patients who have had surgery of the chest or abdomen will be NPO in the period immediately following surgery. Sustenance is reintroduced gradually, as the patient's condition improves. The usual sequence is:
   a. **NPO.** Until signs of bowel function, such as bowel sounds and flatulence, return.
   b. **Clear Liquids.** These include transparent or translucent liquids or semiliquids, such as water, thin broth, apple juice, or gelatin.
   c. **Full Liquids.** The above, plus milk, yogurt, and thicker soups.
   d. **Regular.** See p. 85.
4. Patients may be unable to take oral medicines after surgery. Alternatives include:
   - **Topical Administration.** Nitroglycerin and clonidine can be given topically to treat hypertension. Fentanyl can be given topically for analgesia.
   - **IM Administration.** Especially useful for analgesics, such as morphine and hydromorphone. A nonsteroidal anti-inflammatory drug, ketorolac, has recently become popular for IM use.
   - **SC Administration.** Opioid analgesics as above, as well as insulin.
   - **IV Administration.** Many cardiovascular medications, such as propranolol, metoprolol, atenolol, verapamil, diltiazem, and enalapril, can be given IV. However, their duration of action is short, and they must be given frequently.
   - **Rectal Administration.** Useful for acetaminophen, as well as morphine and hydromorphone.
   - **Sublingual.** Useful primarily for nitroglycerin. Nifedipine SL is sometimes used but is not rec-

ommended since it can cause precipitate falls in blood pressure.

Prescriptions

1. A prescription is an instruction to a pharmacist for an outpatient medication.
2. The blank prescription form looks like this.

Argus Bigwig, M.D.
525 East 68th Street
New York, NY 10021

(212) 555-1234

DEA # ________
LIC. # 555555

NAME ______________________________ AGE ______

ADDRESS ______________________________ DATE __________

____

THIS PRESCRIPTION WILL BE FILLED GENERICALLY
UNLESS PRESCRIBER WRITES 'd a w' IN THE BOX BELOW

Refill ______ times

NR _____ Label _____

Dispense as written

Features include:

- The doctor's name, which must be imprinted (not handwritten) on the form.
- The doctor's license number.
- A blank for the Drug Enforcement Administration (DEA) number. The DEA number is required for all controlled substances, usually including narcotics, sedatives, hypnotics, and other drugs that are susceptible to abuse (androgenic hormones, sympathomimetics). Many states require special prescription blanks for most of these medications anyway. The DEA number should be written on prescriptions for these medications but not for other medications. (The fewer people who know your DEA number, the better.)
- Various blank spaces as depicted.

3. **Refills.** A medication can be refilled zero to six times, or sometimes more. Many pharmacies will limit refills to a year supply, or sometimes less. Refills are convenient for chronic medications. A few caveats:
   - Refills should not be used for one-time medications.
   - Refills usually cannot be written for controlled substances. This varies from state to state
   - Be wary of providing refills for patients who might abuse medication or for patients with poor follow-up patterns
4. **NR.** If the prescription form has a space for NR, it means "No Refill."
5. **Brand or Generic.** All medicines have two names: a *chemical* (or *generic*) name assigned in the development process, and a *brand* name assigned by a manufacturer. *Generic substitution* means that a pharmacist may use any manufacturer of the medication you order. The generic version of a medicine has the identical active compound as the brand name version. It may differ in production technique, binders, dissolv-

ing agents, coatings, etc. The brand name version is usually more expensive than the generic version.

State laws uniformly require that a pharmacist use the least expensive version of a medicine, unless the physician specifically indicates that this may not be done. Prescription blanks have a means of indicating that the physician requires the brand name version. Options are "Do Not Substitute" or "Dispense as Written (DAW)."

Generic substitution does NOT mean that the pharmacist may substitute a similar medicine of the same class.

Most generic versions of medications are therapeutically equivalent to the brand name versions. You *might* wish to require the brand name version for certain medications for which the therapeutic window is narrow, or for which a precise blood level is crucial. These include warfarin, digoxin, and anticonvulsants.

Patients will sometimes request brand names under the mistaken impression that more expensive means better. You should try to resist this pressure by explaining generic substitution.

6. **Label.** Some prescription blanks offer you a choice of whether the medication is to be labeled or not. This blank should virtually always be checked.
7. How to write a prescription (see example)
   - Write the patient's name and the date at the top of the form. Address and age need not be written.
   - The prescription consists of three lines:
     - Name of the medication and tablet size
     - Dispense: [the quantity you wish dispensed, e.g., number of pills]
     - Sig: [how the medicine is to be taken—an abbreviation of the Latin *signa*, meaning *write*]
   - Sign your name

     All prescriptions by medical students must be co-signed by a physician.

- Indicate refill instructions (and label instructions, if necessary)
- If you wish to prohibit generic substitution, indicate as required by your state's regulations.

Argus Bigwig, M.D.
525 East 68th Street
New York, NY 10021

(212) 555-1234
DEA # ________
LIC. # 555555

NAME *Clint Bongo* AGE ______
ADDRESS ______________________ DATE *7/14/95*

Amoxicillin 250 mg
Disp: 30
Sig: 1 PO TID for 10 days

Argus Bigwig, MD

THIS PRESCRIPTION WILL BE FILLED GENERICALLY
UNLESS PRESCRIBER WRITES 'd a w' IN THE BOX BELOW

Refill ______ times

NR ✓ Label ✓

Dispense as written

8. Additional points
   - Be wary of dispensing large amounts, or numerous refills, of potentially toxic medications. This

is especially true of antidepressants, sedatives, and narcotics.

- Remember to check the size of pills. A patient who receives metoprolol 25 mg PO qD in the hospital will need 50-mg tablets, $\frac{1}{2}$ PO qD at home.
- Check bottle sizes for liquids and the like.

CHAPTER 7

Procedures

Performing Procedures

1. A medical procedure is a mechanical intervention made on a patient's body. The procedures most often performed by students and interns include venipuncture, intravenous catheter placement, arterial puncture, central venous catheter placement (central line), lumbar puncture, thoracentesis, and paracentesis.
2. These are generally performed at the patient's bedside. In some instances, a special procedure room is used.
3. The sequence for learning a new procedure is:
   a. Familiarize yourself with the indications, contraindications, and complications—described in the next section.
   b. Ask your supervisor to describe the steps.
   c. Observe a competent operator when he or she performs the procedure. You may wish to observe several times before attempting it yourself.
   d. When you feel certain that you understand what to do, ask your supervisor if it is appropriate that you perform the procedure on a patient. The first time, or several times, that you perform a procedure, it should be under the direct supervision of a competent operator.
   e. When you are capable of performing the procedure under direct supervision, ask your super-

visor if it is appropriate that you perform the procedure under indirect supervision; that is, without the supervisor being physically present in the room.

4. Always check with a supervisor before performing a procedure.

Indications and Contraindications

1. All procedures, as well as all treatments and tests, have indications and contraindications.
2. An *indication* is a reason to perform a procedure.

Examples

- Coronary artery disease involving three vessels is an indication for coronary artery bypass grafting.
- Acute pulmonary embolus is an indication for intravenous heparin.

3. A *contraindication* is a reason *not* to perform a procedure.

An *absolute contraindication* is when present, the procedure should not be done.

Examples

- Acute myocardial infarction is an absolute contraindication to elective cholecystectomy.
- Actively bleeding duodenal ulcer is an absolute contraindication to thrombolytic therapy.

A *relative contraindication* is when present, the procedure should not be undertaken lightly; risk is increased. The procedure may be performed if necessary and if the increased risk is taken into consideration.

Example

- Past history of duodenal ulcer is a relative contraindication to aspirin therapy.

Complications

1. A complication is an adverse effect of a procedure, treatment, or other intervention.
2. Distinguish:
   - An expected adverse outcome. This type of complication may be frequent but generally implies mild consequences.

     Examples

     - Mild local discomfort after lumbar puncture
     - Tachycardia after treatment with nitroglycerin

   - An adverse outcome that is known to occur in some proportion of patients, but that cannot be predicted for the individual patient. This type of complication generally carries a low but nonzero frequency.

     Examples

     - Headache after lumbar puncture
     - Stroke during carotid endarterectomy

   - An unexpected, unpredictable adverse outcome. The frequency of this type of complication should be very low.

     Example

     - Death after lumbar puncture
3. All procedures and interventions carry a risk of complication. The physician should understand the potential complications of a procedure and should discuss them with the patient.
4. **Risk and Benefit.** The physician and the patient must decide whether the potential benefit from a medical intervention justifies the potential risk. Both parties are involved in the decision-making process. As a general rule, the physician presents each of the options to the patient and discusses their potential benefits and risks. It is the patient

who ultimately makes the final decision in most cases.

Informed Consent

1. All patients should understand the reasons for doing a procedure and the potential complications of the procedure.
2. These should be discussed with the patient. The physician is responsible for ensuring that the patient understands the risks, benefits, and potential complications of a procedure.
3. This discussion should be documented in the medical record, especially for procedures with significant risk. The format for documenting consent is described in Chapter 4, "Writing Notes."
4. All surgical procedures, and many other invasive procedures, require that a patient sign a form that documents his or her consen

Procedures That Require Signed Consent	Procedures That Do Not Require Signed Consent
All operations	Physical examination
Central venous catheter	Venipuncture
Arterial catheter	Intravenous catheter (peripheral)
Thoracentesis	Arterial puncture (varies)
Paracentesis	Nasogastric tube
Lumbar puncture	Bandage or dressing
Suturing	Plain radiographs, CT, or ultrasound
Reduction of fractures	Administration of ordinary medications
Fiberoptic procedures	Specimen collection
Endoscopies	
Administration of IV contrast dye	
MRI	
Cancer chemotherapy	
Experimental treatments	
Participation in research	

5. When a patient is unable to comprehend the ramifications of the procedure and of consent, the physician is responsible for obtaining consent from another party. The question of who may make medical decisions for another is regulated by state law.
   - If an adult patient is competent to make decisions, the patient makes his or her own decisions. For a child, the parent or next nearest relative is responsible for making decisions. Note that a family does not override the wishes of an elderly or sick patient if the patient is competent.
   - **Health Care Proxy.** In some states, a person may name another person as the health care agent. The agent is authorized to make all medical decisions for the patient *if* the patient is unable to make his or her own decisions. If the patient is able to make decisions, the agent has no authority. The patient must choose an agent while still competent.
   - If there is no proxy, decisions may be made by the following persons, in order of authority:
     - A court-appointed guardian—often an attorney or hospital administrator
     - Spouse
     - Adult child
     - Sibling
     - Parent
     - Other close relative
     - Close friend
6. Consent is implied for emergency, life-saving treatment, if there is no opportunity to obtain specific consent

   Example

   > Signed consent is ordinarily required for endotracheal intubation. If a person suffers respiratory arrest and is unconscious, intubation should be performed at once, without obtaining signed consent—unless the patient (or agent) has formally indicated that this is not desired.

Common Procedures

Venipuncture

1. *Indication:*	To remove a sample of venous blood for testing
2. *Contraindications:*	Infection of overlying skin Lymphedema of extremity Ipsilateral lymph node dissection Intravenous line distal to site
3. *Complications:*	Infection Thrombosis Laceration of vessel Bleeding

Intravenous Catheter Placement

1. *Indication:*	To administer intravenous medication, fluid, or blood product
2. *Contraindications:*	Infection of overlying skin Lymphedema of extremity Ipsilateral lymph node dissection
3. *Complications:*	Infection Thrombosis Laceration of vessel Bleeding Air embolization

Arterial Puncture

1. *Indication:*	To remove a sample of arterial blood for testing
2. *Contraindications:*	Infection of overlying skin Lymphedema of extremity Ipsilateral lymph node dissection Arterial insufficiency

3. *Complications:* Infection
Thrombosis
Laceration of vessel
Bleeding
Atheromatous embolization

Central Venous Catheter

1. *Indications:* To administer medication, fluid or blood product into the central circulation
To measure central venous pressure
2. *Contraindications:* Infection of overlying skin
3. *Complications:* Infection
Thrombosis
Laceration of vessel
Bleeding
Pneumothorax (for internal jugular and subclavian catheters)
Air embolization

Lumbar Puncture

1. *Indications:* To remove a sample of cerebral spinal fluid (CSF) for testing
To administer medication or contrast material into the CSF
2. *Contraindications:* Infection of overlying skin
Increased intracranial pressure (relative)
3. *Complications:* Cellulitis
Meningitis
Headache
Bleeding
Arachnoiditis
Radiculopathy

Thoracentesis

1. *Indication:* To remove fluid from a pleural effusion, for diagnostic or therapeutic purposes
2. *Contraindications:* Infection of overlying skin
   Nonlayering fluid (relative)
   Severe emphysematous changes (relative)
3. *Complications:* Infection
   Bleeding
   Pneumothorax
   Hemothorax

Paracentesis

1. *Indication:* To remove ascitic fluid for diagnostic or therapeutic purposes
2. *Contraindications:* Infection of overlying skin
   Hypotension (relative)
   Severe bowel distention
3. *Complications:* Infection
   Bleeding
   Hypotension
   Lacerated or punctured organ
   Perforated abdominal viscus

CHAPTER 8

Preventing Nosocomial Infection

General Principles

1. *Nosocomial infection* refers to a contagious illness that is contracted in a hospital—or, by extension, in other clinical settings. Infections may be spread among any of four parties: patients, visitors, the public, and health-care workers. Proper infection control measures by health-care workers can prevent the transmission of these diseases.
2. Each infectious disease has a characteristic route of transmission. There are four main means of transmitting infectious diseases.
   - **Contact Route.** The organism is spread by touch. This may be:
     - Direct contact—for example, touching the patient
     - Indirect contact—for example, touching contaminated bed linens
     - Droplet spread—for example, cough
   - **Vehicle Route.** The organism is spread by a contaminated substance, such as:
     - Contaminated food—for example, *Salmonella* enteritis

    - Contaminated water—for example, cholera
    - Contaminated drugs—for example, bacterial infection of eyedrops
    - Contaminated blood—for example, hepatitis B
  - **Airborne Route.** The organism is carried in the air.
    - For example, histoplasmosis
  - **Vector Route.** The organism is transmitted via passage in another animal.
    - For example, malaria, Lyme disease
3. Infectious diseases occur differently among different persons.
   - **Prevalence.** A disease may occur more frequently in certain groups. For example, tuberculosis occurs more frequently among the homeless than in others. These persons are more likely than others to introduce an infection into the hospital.
   - **Susceptibility.** A person may be more susceptible than are others to certain infections. For example, a person with leukemia is more susceptible to sepsis with *Pseudomonas*. These persons are more likely than others to acquire an infection in the hospital.
4. By understanding routes of transmission and variable host conditions, health-care workers can block transmission and prevent disease.
5. A health-care worker who becomes sick should avoid infecting others. Skin wounds must be covered at all times. For mild cough, a mask should be worn for patient contact. For moderate or severe cough, one should not have contact with patients. In addition, one must not have contact with patients if one has any of the following:
   - Diarrhea
   - Any febrile illness
   - Any other highly contagious illness, such as strep throat, viral exanthems, scabies, pneumonia, etc.

Universal Precautions

1. The concept of *Universal Precautions* assumes that all persons may be potentially infected with blood-borne pathogens. The concept was designed by the Centers for Disease Control to minimize the risk of exposure for health-care workers to infectious blood and body fluids. Its basic tenet is that, since it is impossible to know in advance which patient has a blood-borne disease, one should treat all patients as though such a disease might be present.
2. *Handwashing* before and after contact with each patient is the single most important means of preventing the spread of infection. Washing the hands is mandatory. The procedure is simple.
   a. Wet hands.
   b. Apply antimicrobial soap.
   c. Wash vigorously for at least 10 seconds.
   d. Rinse thoroughly, with the hands pointing down.
   e. Dry thoroughly.
   f. Use the paper towel to turn off the faucet. This prevents contaminating your clean hands with any organisms that might adhere to the faucet.
3. *Protective attire* is used to prevent contact between the worker's skin or mucous membranes, and patient blood or body fluids. Most protective attire is disposable. All disposable attire is used once, for one patient, and then discarded.
   - *Gloves* are worn as follows:
     - Whenever contact with blood or body fluids is expected
     - For contact with items contaminated with blood or body fluids
     - For all blood drawing
     - For all procedures within the body, such as the examination of the mouth, rectum, or vagina
     - For all handling of patient specimens

- For all contact with patients who have diseases transmitted by direct contact, such as Methcillin-resistant *Staphylococcus aureus*
- Whenever the worker has a cut or abraded skin

Gloves need not be sterile for most uses. *Sterile gloves* are used for surgical procedures and for certain other invasive procedures.

- *Gowns* are worn when:
  - One's clothing may be contaminated by blood or body fluids
  - The patient has a disease transmitted by direct contact, such as pseudomembranous colitis

  Highly moisture-resistant gowns are used for procedures especially likely to spread fluids, such as endoscopic gastrostomy in a patient with a bleeding esophageal varix. Sterile gowns are worn in surgery.
- *Masks and protective eyewear* are used to protect the face and eyes. These are worn whenever blood or body fluids might be splashed into the face (e.g., during fiberoptic bronchoscopy). Any health-care worker who has a cough should also wear a mask to avoid infecting others.

4. *Waste disposal* is an important feature of infection control. Medical waste that is contaminated with patient blood or fluids is treated specially and is placed in special waste containers. Cancer chemotherapeutic agents and radioactive materials also receive special treatment. Each hospital and ambulatory facility develops regulations governing the handling of such materials; you will become familiar with these for each facility at which you train.
   - All *sharp disposable instruments*, including needles, syringes, and blades, are placed in puncture-resistant containers. These should be located in all patient care areas. Guidelines for handling "sharps" include the following:

  - Needles should not be recapped.
  - Syringes, with or without needles, should be discarded intact into a sharps container
  - Tubing connected to a needle is cut above the level of contamination and placed into a sharps container
  - Sharps should be placed immediately into an appropriate container—not left sitting for eventual disposal.
- *Body secretions* should be discarded in special flushing sinks. All patient care areas should have a utility room, often called the *dirty utility room*, designed for this purpose. Secretions may be discarded in a regular patient toilet, if the patient has a private bathroom. Some centers require that liquid waste be mixed with a disinfectant before disposal.
- *Spills* should be cleaned immediately, using gloves. Materials used to clean spills of blood or body fluids are regarded as contaminated. For certain materials, such as cancer chemotherapeutic agents or radioactive substances, special procedures are used. For extensive spills, the housekeeping department should be notified.

5. *Laboratory specimens* should be labeled immediately after collection and then placed in plastic bags. A second label must sometimes be placed on the outside of the bag. Lids must be secure. If you need to pour specimens from one container to another, do so in the dirty utility room.

Special Isolation

1. Special procedures are employed to prevent the transmission of specific types of diseases.
   - *Enteric precautions* are used for diseases with fecal-to-oral transmission, such as hepatitis A. The patient must have a private bathroom or com-

mode. Dining materials are usually disposable. Energetic handwashing is crucial.

- *Respiratory precautions* are used for diseases potentially transmitted by cough, such as chickenpox. The patient must have a private room and may not leave the room without wearing a mask. Health-care workers must wear masks. In certain situations—especially if tuberculosis is suspected—special particulate filter masks must be worn.
- *Wound and skin precautions* are used for diseases transmitted by direct contact, such as scabies. Gloves and gowns must be worn.
- *Reverse isolation* is used for patients who are especially susceptible to infection, such as those who are immune-compromised from cancer chemotherapy or an inherited immune deficiency. Live plants, uncooked fruit etc. must not be brought into the room. Visitors must wash their hands on entering and leaving the room. Masks are sometimes worn.
- *Unusual precautions* involve strict isolation procedures for highly contagious diseases infrequently encountered, such as plague or kuru.

2. Precautions should be ordered whenever the conditions previously listed are documented *or suspected.* The patient's room should be marked with appropriate labeling. Protective measures must be taken by visitors as well as by medical personnel.

Preventing Injury to Oneself

1. Students and interns can avoid injuring or infecting themselves by using proper technique for examination, surgery, and procedures. Injury with sharp instruments, such as needles and scapels, occurs most commonly when you are in a hurry or are inattentive. Calm, purposeful, methodic technique prevents these injuries.

2. Surgery often brings a large number of hands and instruments to a small space. You can avoid injury by:
   - Keeping extraneous fingers and instruments out of the surgical field
   - Passing instruments to others by offering the handle end
   - Using instruments, rather than the fingers, to hold needles
   - Taking your time
3. Learners are also liable to injure themselves when performing procedures with which they are unfamiliar. You should rehearse the steps of a new procedure before actually performing it. Requesting help or supervision until you are comfortable with a procedure is entirely appropriate.
4. Occasionally, a violent or deranged patient may threaten to injure you. Your options in this instance include restraints, sedation, or security escort. It is not advisable to restrain a violent patient bodily without assistance.
5. If you sustain an *accidental needlestick injury*, or if you have accidental contact with body fluids, the following applies:
   - Wash the exposed area thoroughly.
   - Contact your student or employee health department immediately. All medical schools and hospitals have policies that govern accidental exposures.
   - Seek emergency care, if recommended.

   It may be advisable to check the HIV and hepatitis B status of the patient and yourself. For high-risk exposures, postexposure prophylaxis is sometimes indicated. A tetanus booster is generally recommended if 5 years or more have elapsed since the last booster.

   If you have a significant, unprotected exposure to a patient with tuberculosis, you should contact your student or employee health office on the next working day. PPD testing or chest x-ray is ordinarily recommended about 6 weeks after the exposure. Exposure is considered not to have occurred if the clinician has used a mask appropriately.

6. *Vaccination* is extremely important. For all health-care workers:
   - Hepatitis B vaccine is recommended. There is zero risk of contracting HIV or other diseases from the vaccine.
   - Antibody titres for measles, mumps, and rubella should be drawn, and vaccine should be administered, as needed.
   - Antibody titres for varicella should be drawn. Health-care workers who are not immune to varicella should not care for patients with documented or suspected varicella infection. If an accidental exposure should occur, the worker must usually avoid patient care for a period of quarantine Vaccine is now available.
   - Tetanus immunization should be up to date, implying vaccination every 10 years.
   - Primary immunization for tetanus, diphtheria, pertussis, and polio should be completed.
   - Influenza vaccine should be administered annually, usually in October or November.
7. *PPD testing* should be performed annually—or twice annually, for certain high-risk areas. For persons who have had a positive PPD in the past, periodic chest x-rays are indicated.

Preventing HIV Infection

1. HIV can be transmitted via blood or body secretions. For patients with HIV, the virus has been isolated from virtually every type of body fluid.
2. Nosocomial transmission of HIV may occur by:
   - *Percutaneous exposure*
     - Needlestick

  - Surgical instruments
- *Integument exposure*
  - Eye
  - Mouth
  - Nonintact skin

3. The risk of transmitting HIV varies according to the type of exposure. For percutaneous injuries with a sharp instrument contaminated with HIV, the risk of contracting HIV is estimated to be 0.3%. The risk is higher for deep exposures through hollow-bore needles (such as those used to draw blood or to inject medication) or for actual injections. The greater the bolus of injected material, the higher the risk. The risk is less for superficial exposures by solid needles (such as suture needles). There have been a few anecdotal case reports of transmission via the eye, mouth, or broken skin; the risk of these routes is considered low but not negligible. There have been no cases of transmission through intact skin or aerosol.

   The higher the patient's level of circulating HIV, the greater the risk of transmission in accidental exposures. High blood levels of HIV occur during the initial infection and late in the disease. Levels are low during the asymptomatic phase, then increase as the disease progresses.
4. Nosocomial infection with HIV can be prevented by adhering to Universal Precautions. It is crucial to foster a safe workplace environment, as previously outlined. However, it is also important to recognize the many situations in which HIV cannot be transmitted. If neither the patient nor the clinician has open skin wounds, gloves are not necessary for routine physical examination or interviewing. Masks are not needed unless pulmonary tuberculosis is suspected. Exaggerating the use of masks and gloves can make the patient feel like a pariah, while betraying ignorance of disease transmission.

5. All persons, including those with HIV, are entitled to the same type and quality of care. To avoid patients with HIV is completely inexcusable and should not be tolerated. It jeopardizes the basic tenets of compassionate care and threatens the heart of medicine.
6. Prophylactic AZT after accidental exposure to HIV is a controversial issue. Arguments in favor of taking AZT after an exposure are as follows:
   - It appears beneficial in experimental retroviral inoculation of cats and mice.
   - No serious side effects have been reported in health-care workers.
   - It is recommended by the National Institutes of Health.

   Arguments against taking AZT after an exposure are as follows:
   - There are no data in humans.
   - No benefit has been observed in experimental retroviral inoculation of primates.
   - The long-term side effects are unknown.

   The decision must thus be made on a case-by-case basis. Consulting with a subspecialist in HIV disease may be helpful.

CHAPTER 9

Relations with Patients

Principles

1. Medicine is above all a profession of principles. While almost everything we understand about human physiology and disease has changed since the era of Hippocrates, the principles espoused by his school have remained remarkably durable. You know, too, that many of the biomedical facts you have learned in your training will be revised or discarded during the course of your career; the principles of the doctor-patient relationship will stand you in good stead.
2. The two hallmark principles of the doctor-patient relationship are dedication and respect. *Dedication* means that you will devote yourself, to the best of your ability, to the good of your patients. *Respect* means that you will treat all patients, and indeed all others whom you encounter in the practice of medicine, as humans like yourself—with concerns, ideas, emotions, and desires like your own.
3. These two basic principles have a variety of interpersonal, ethical, and medicolegal ramifications.

Interpersonal Relations

1. **Listen.** When patients are surveyed, their most frequently cited cause for dissatisfaction with their medical care is a sense of inadequate communication. While the physician has a problem-solving agenda that requires him or her to probe for information and pinpoint facts, the patient also needs to talk and to be heard. In fact, sympathetically inviting the patient to speak often provides the best history and confers a therapeutic benefit as well.
2. **Care.** Francis Weld Peabody: "One of the essential qualities of the clinician is interest in humanity, for the secret of the care of the patient is in caring for the patient."[1] What Peabody means in this famous dictum is that good patient care is the natural outcome of interest in the patient's well-being.
3. **Explain.** While few patients have the benefit of advanced biomedical education, most can understand what is happening to them medically. It is your responsibility to explain their medical condition to them in terms that they can understand. This is not difficult if you make it a priority.

   Adjusting the discussion to the patient's level of understanding is important. As you begin to talk, the patient's degree of familiarity with medical terms and principles will become apparent. You will need to modify your language accordingly, avoiding both excessive simplicity and excessive complication. Jargon and doublespeak should be avoided.
4. **Understand.** Put the patient's illness and health in

---

[1]Peabody, FW: The care of the patient. JAMA 1927;88: 877–882.

the context of the patient's life as a whole. Each patient has a personal life, needs, aspirations, emotions, etc. Most have jobs and families. Understanding these aspects of the patient's life will help you to participate in the healing process.

5. **Be Patient.** Remember that patients feel unwell. They are anxious, uncomfortable, worried, disrupted, out of their element, and disconnected from their usual support systems. They may be grappling with major life issues, including death. These concerns outweigh whatever you may be feeling in terms of being tired, bedraggled, pressured, or irritable.
6. **Be Honest.** If you don't know the answer to a patient's question, say that you don't know. Also make it clear that you will find out the answer and communicate it to the patient.
7. **Find Out.** If your patient has (or may have) aortic stenosis or familial Mediterranean fever, make it a point to become the week's expert on aortic stenosis or familial Mediterranean fever.
8. **Respect.** It warrants repetition. Terms such as "gomer," "dirtball," and worse have no place in patient communication and should not be tolerated. Treat the patient as you would like to be treated.
9. **Addressing Patients.** Adult patients should be addressed formally as Mr. Smith, Ms. Jones, Mrs. Doe, Dr. Roe, etc. Children can be addressed by their first names. Be sure you know the patient's name before you enter the examination or hospital room, so that you can greet him or her cordially without checking the chart or their nameband. When you have known a patient for some time and have established a good relation, you can use your judgment about using first names. When in doubt, the formal address is better.
10. **Attending to Your Family Members.** This should

be avoided, if possible. They will often call on you regarding medical conditions. While you can help to guide them through the system, it is inadvisable to render medical opinions or to provide their care yourself. You cannot hope to be objective in attending to family members, and you or they may feel uncomfortable in some of the more personal aspects of medical interaction. Further, the therapeutic benefit of the doctor-patient relation itself, when it functions well, may not occur if superseded by a familial relationship. Your most important role in the illness of a relative may be to be a good son or daughter or nephew, rather than a physician.

Some physicians will feel conflicts in providing care to personal friends. If you feel that you cannot evaluate the patient objectively, or that your judgment seems clouded, discuss your feeling with the friend and consider referring them to another physician.

A corollary of these principles is to avoid prescribing medications on a casual basis to family members, friends, or coworkers. If acquaintances request treatment from you, they should have the same history and physical examination that you would offer a stranger—certainly not less.

11. **Pay Attention to How a Patient Makes You Feel.** Your emotional response can be most informative. A personal feeling of unease could come from some aspect of the patient, or from some aspect of yourself.

Patient Causes of Physician Unease

- **Situational.** Anxiety, pain, and fear can cause the patient to be irritable, querulous, or mistrustful.
- **Personality and Personality Disorders.** The patient may be constitutionally anxious, aggressive, hostile, evasive, seductive, or passive. The

borderline personality disorder, characterized by difficulties in forming personal relations, can be especially trying.

- **Socialization Skills.** There are implicit conventions for interactions between physicians and patients, with stereotypical modes of address, speech, dress, and behavior. A patient who does not "play the part" may not know the expected role or may decide not to play it.
- **Psychosis.** Psychosis, especially in schizophrenia, creates in others a powerful sense of disconnectedness. If a patient makes you feel that you are not establishing personal contact, consider this diagnosis.

Physician Causes of Physician Unease

- You may feel uncomfortable with some aspect of the medical history or examination. This applies especially for the gynecologic, urologic, and sexual components of the evaluation; and for questions regarding drugs, alcohol, and personal stressors.
- You may feel uncomfortable with particular kinds of patients. Perhaps they remind you of a relative or of some aspect of your personal life.
- You may feel attracted to a patient. This is normal but should be deflected and relegated to a strictly professional relation.
- You may feel repulsed by a patient—because of a physical deformity, severe injury, or some other attribute. To which Hippocrates rejoins,[2] "The medical man sees terrible sights, touches unpleasant things, and the misfortunes of others bring a harvest of sorrows that are peculiarly his; but the sick by means of the art rid them-

---

[2]Hippocrates: Breaths. In Hippocrates, with an English Translation by W.H.S. Jones, vol. 2. Cambridge, MA, Harvard University Press, 1923, p 227.

selves of the worst of evils, disease, suffering, pain and death."

- You may feel uncertain in an area of knowledge. This can be remedied with a few minutes of study.
- You may feel unable to help a patient. Patients with severe or untreatable illnesses often report that other persons, including physicians, shun them. Yet the physician has an important role in treating all patients, guarding against (or masking) personal discouragement or hopelessness.
- You may yourself be bringing personal, external stress to the doctor-patient relation.
- You may yourself have a personality disorder or an ineffective socialization skill.

The first group tells you about the patient; the second about yourself. In the latter case, thoughtful introspection can help you to channel your behavior along professional lines. You are not expected to exclude or to suppress your personal makeup in interacting with patients; indeed, the doctor-patient relation depends on your expressing your own character. However, professionalism mandates that you keep your purely private issues in the background, and that you direct yourself to the patient's needs.

Ethical Responsibilities

1. **Confidentiality.** This is of the utmost importance. You should discuss a patient only with another health-care provider, and only for the purpose of improving care. You should not discuss patient information in any public place, such as an elevator, cafeteria, hallway, sidewalk, or any other place where the conversation might be overheard. You should reveal neither that a celebrity was in the hospital nor that you saw a neighbor in your office.

   Hippocrates: "And whatsoever I shall see or hear

in the course of my profession, as well as outside my profession in my intercourse with men, if it be what should not be published abroad, I will never divulge, holding such things to be holy secrets."[3]

Be wary of assuming that a patient wants you to discuss medical information with, or in front of, a spouse or other family member. It is best to ask the patient, preferably in private. When family members or acquaintances are present, you can ask them to leave for a few moments while you talk with the patient.

There may be a temptation to peruse the chart of a patient whose name you recognize, or to discuss their case with one of their doctors. This temptation should be resisted. You really do not need to know about the senator's gallbladder or the nurse's hysterectomy.

2. **Being There.** The patient must know that you, or a substitute, are available to attend them when circumstances demand. This means:
   - That you can be reached—by telephone, beeper, or other mechanism
   - That the patient knows how to reach you
   - That you will respond promptly
   - That you can arrange for the patient to be evaluated promptly
   - That there is a mechanism to provide coverage at all times: 24 hours a day, 365 days a year
3. **Beneficence.** This means that you act in the patient's best interest. This is not to say that the doctor-patient relation is not mutually beneficial. The physician receives insight, education, compensation, and a privileged place in society. Yet these

[3]Hippocrates: The Oath. In Hippocrates, with an English Translation by W.H.S. Jones, Vol. 1, Cambridge, MA, Harvard University Press, 1923, p 301.

must be held secondary to what is best for the patient.

Your purpose in practicing medicine is to help your patients, not to enrich, amuse, or magnify yourself. A patient may call when you would rather be sleeping; another may develop an emergency when you had a tennis court reserved. Your response should be to take a deep breath and to take care of them.

4. **Primum Non Nocere.** This well-known phrase is a Latin translation from the Hippocratic Oath that means, "First, do no harm." The maxim acknowledges the imperfect state of medical knowledge and implies that, whatever you attempt to do for the patient, the minimum requirement is to try to avoid injuring them. Many medical procedures subject the patient to risk; but it is imperative to confer the minimum possible risk. In particular, unproved or improbable treatments should not be recommended, and dangerous plans should not be recommended unless there is a substantial possibility of success. Medical history is filled with examples of painful or harmful treatments that were eloquently espoused by leaders in the field, enthusiastically applied by practitioners, and otherwise fruitless.
5. **Being Knowledgeable.** You are expected to bring the state of the art to each patient encounter. This means that you must know medicine well, that you must stay current, and that you will apply your knowledge conscientiously. One corollary is that you will inform yourself when you are unsure. Another (also named in the Hippocratic Oath) is that you will refer to more expert physicians when you reach your personal limit of expertise.
6. **Self-determination. This** means that the patient has a right to decide his or her own course, including making medical decisions. It is for the patient, not the doctor, to decide what is best. The clinician

must make every effort to see to it that the patient understands the medical issues, the choices at hand, and the likely outcomes of each choice. The physician must provide the patient with the information necessary to make an informed choice.

7. **Fairness.** This means that all patients should receive the same medical care. Issues of payment, insurance, gender, race, sexual orientation, religion, or any other personal attributes should not affect your behavior or care.

Legal Responsibilities

1. Many of the physician's legal responsibilities are the logical extensions of the ethical issues previously outlined. There are statutes regarding confidentiality and nonstatutory rules regarding patient access to physicians, acting within one's areas of knowledge, and avoiding conflicts of interest.
2. **Documentation.** Physicians are required to maintain written records of their interactions with patients. These include complete and accurate accounts of the medical history, examinations, laboratory data, radiographic and pathologic reports, and conversations with the patient or with others. Documents must be made available to others at the request of the patient and only with the patient's express consent.

   The medical record is a legal document. Once written, it cannot be altered in any way. If your opinion changes, write your new interpretation as a new entry into the record.

   As was discussed in Chapter 4, "Writing Notes," the medical record should consist of objective facts and reasoned interpretations of them. It should not contain unsubstantiated opinions.

   Rules of confidentiality also apply to written records. No part of a medical record may be divulged to another party without the consent of the patient.

3. **Informed Consent.** Nothing should be done to a patient without his or her consent. Informed consent has two aspects.
   - The patient must understand the reasons for the recommended action, the potential risks, and the potential benefits.
   - The patient must agree to undertake the action.

   The clinician must ensure that both of these aspects have been discussed, and that the patient understands what is at stake if he or she wishes to proceed. This discussion should be documented in the medical record.

   Consent is implied for life-threatening emergencies. For example, if a person is found unconscious after being struck by a car, it is assumed that he or she would consent to being brought to the hospital by ambulance and undergoing treatment. However, consent cannot be assumed if the person is able to understand the situation and to express his or her wishes.

   Obtaining and documenting consent is discussed more fully in Chapter 4, "Writing Notes," and in Chapter 7, "Procedures."
4. **Competence.** Competence refers to a person's ability to make decisions. A person may not be competent to make decisions if:
   - He or she is a minor.
   - He or she is unable to understand the risks, benefits, and ramifications of a medical procedure or treatment. One might be unable to understand such matters because of low intelligence or altered mental status. Altered mental status, in turn, might occur because of delirium, psychosis, encephalopathy, stroke, intoxication, drug effect, dementia, or another process affecting the brain.

- He or she has psychiatric illness. For example, a patient with severe depression might not be competent to make decisions regarding the risks and benefits of treatment.

A patient is assumed competent until proven otherwise. This means that, if you have accepted a patient's consent for a procedure, you have inferred that the patient is competent. It is not reasonable to question competence only when the patient refuses a procedure that the doctor wishes to perform.

The ultimate authority in deciding competence is the court system. The finding that a patient is able to understand the ramifications of medical procedures can be made by a physician; a neurologist or a psychiatrist is often asked to make this determination.

5. **Advance Directives.** Persons have the opportunity to anticipate what their wishes regarding their medical care might be in the event that they become unable to express their wishes. This indication of one's future wishes is called an *advance directive.* The advance directive allows the patient to indicate what medical procedures he or she would want to undergo under various circumstances.

An advance directive could indicate any type of medical care but is typically employed in matters of cardiopulmonary resuscitation, advanced life support, mechanical ventilator support, renal dialysis, and artificial nutrition. For example, a person might assert that, in the event of cardiopulmonary arrest, he or she would not wish to undergo cardiopulmonary resuscitation. Another might state that he or she would not wish to undergo tracheal intubation, or hemodialysis, under any circumstances.

The advance directive is best written down, either as a formal legal document or in the medical record. It is essential that the patient be competent to make decisions at the time the directive is formulated. While anyone can make directives, they are most appropriate for persons with serious progressive illness or for the elderly.

6. **Health Care Proxy.** Health care proxy is available in some states and allows a person to name another person as the health care agent. The agent is authorized to make all medical decisions for the patient *if* the patient is unable to make his or her own decisions. If the patient is able to make decisions, the agent has no authority. The patient must choose an agent while still competent. This is discussed further in Chapter 7, "Procedures."
7. **DNR.** DNR refers to "Do Not Resuscitate." DNR is a type of advance directive. It means specifically that the patient does not wish to undergo cardiopulmonary resuscitation in the event of cardiopulmonary arrest. Cardiopulmonary resuscitation in this context means chest compression, artificial ventilation, tracheal intubation, electrical cardioversion or defibrillation, and the use of cardiovascular pressors. If a patient is competent to make decisions, he or she decides whether to elect DNR status; if the patient is not competent, the health care agent makes this decision.

   The clinician is responsible for discussing DNR status with patients. This discussion, and the resultant decision, should be documented in the medical record. Many states require that a specific form be completed. The attending physician has the ultimate responsibility for DNR and must sign the appropriate documents.
8. **Persons Who Do Not Speak English.** These people are entitled to the same medical care as everyone else. Obtaining a translator is essential. If your foreign language skills are rudimentary, it is often better to find a fluent translator than to

struggle clumsily to obtain a medical history, where precise description is so important. Ideally, the patient will bring a friend or family member to translate; this should be encouraged. Alternatively, bilingual hospital staff may be available. As a last resort, a commercial translation service is available by telephone for a great number of foreign languages. Not understanding the English language, in the absence of other problems in competence, does not make a person incompetent. The clinician must make every effort to obtain a translator.

9. **Research.** A patient receives care based on the belief that the doctor is recommending the course of action that seems best for the patient. The premise of clinical research is that the best course of action is unknown and warrants investigation. A physician must not involve a patient in research without express consent. Consent for research involves the same discussion of risks and benefits as consent for medical procedures.
10. **Standard of Care.** This means that a physician should provide, as a minimum, the level of care that is generally accepted and provided in the community. For example, the standard of care for an acute myocardial infarction is hospitalization with cardiac monitoring. You may feel strongly that gargling with garlic is preferable to the conventional plan, but this is not the standard of care.

CHAPTER 10

Being Effective: Goals and Skills

A Day in the Life

1. A typical day's schedule on medicine, pediatrics, or neurology runs as follows:

7:00 AM	See your patients on your own; check vital signs and major events; focused exam. This process may need to begin earlier.
7:15 AM	Morning Rounds.
8:00 AM	Work Rounds.
10:00 AM	Chores—Review x-rays; make sure that blood tests have been drawn; check charts for recommendations; order/schedule diagnostic tests; perform procedures; discuss details with patients.
11:00 AM	Attending Rounds.
12:00 noon	Conference. This may occur at any time of the day but often occurs at lunch; bringing a sandwich is usually considered legitimate.
1:00 PM	Chores. This is usually a good time to write progress notes. You may also see ambulatory patients once or twice a week. There may be new admissions for you.

4:00 PM	"Chart Rounds."
5:30 PM	Sign-Out Rounds.
6:00 PM	Go home. Before you do, always make sure that (1) there are no unattended issues for your patients, and (2) you have checked their most recent vital signs and evaluated any significant changes.

2. A typical day's schedule in surgery, ob/gyn, and other surgical specialties is as follows:

6:00 AM	See your patients on your own; check vital signs and major events; focused exam. This may need to begin earlier.
6:15 AM	Work Rounds.
7:00 AM	Surgery or chores. The team typically breaks up at this point. Some are assigned to perform and assist in surgery; others attend to chores.
12:00 noon	Conference.
1:00 PM	Surgery or chores.
5:30 PM	Sign-Out Rounds.
6:00 PM	Go home.

On Call

1. Being on call means that a subset of the team remains in the hospital while others have gone home.
2. You have two main responsibilities while on call: to admit new patients, and to take care of any problems that might arise in patients on your team.
3. Keys to being effective on call:
   - Make sure that you have an accurate *sign-out* from each of the other caregivers. It should be written and contain meaningful information. Planning in advance for possible contingencies, like fever or chest pain, is helpful.
   - Know which of the patients have DNR status.

- Take care of yourself. This helps you keep well, manage stress, and avoid fatigue and irritability. You should eat meals and drink fluids during the on-call period. If there is time to sleep at night, use it. Calling a friend, spouse, or significant other can help.
- Take care of the patients. Resist the temptation to minimize or to ignore new symptoms or findings.
- See new admissions as early as possible, in the emergency department if necessary.
- Perform diagnostic tests and procedures as early as possible. This allows you to interpret results while there is still time to act on them.
- Avoid performing elective procedures at night, when there is less backup in case of complications.
- Listen to the nurses; they know many of the patients better than you do.
- If a nurse calls you to evaluate a new problem, respond promptly.
- Answer pages immediately.
- Visit each nursing station periodically, and ask if there are any problems. This lets the nurses know that you are available and intend to take care of matters.
- Check vital signs periodically, ideally for all patients under your care.
- Know who the unstable patients are and check in on them periodically.
- Don't hesitate to ask for help. You must know your level of competence and seek someone more experienced when necessary.

Being an Effective Physician-in-Training

1. Take care of your patients. This means:
   - Being the doctor.

    - Understanding each patient's case and situation, and providing treatment, to the best of your ability.
2. Learn. This means:
    - Reading up on your patients' medical conditions.
    - Attending conferences and tutorial sessions.
    - Checking when you don't know—by asking or reading.
3. Play your role in the team. This means:
    - Consuming a fair share of the educational resources.
    - Chores.
    - Behaving conscientiously: being there and being there well.
    - Communicating: with the patient, with the family, with other caregivers, and with a supervising physician.
4. Tips for being effective:
    - Know your patients.
    - **Macromanagement.** Try to get the big picture for each patient. What is the essence of the illness, where is it going, is it likely to improve or worsen? What should the patient expect? How does the illness fit into the patient's life?
    - **Micromanagement.** Keep on top of details. What is the most recent condition of the patient's symptoms, physical findings, and laboratory data?
    - Review data yourself. Look at each physical finding, at each x-ray, at the blood smear, rather than depending on someone else's description.
    - Think for yourself. You will learn the most, and help your patient the most, if you develop your own interpretation and plan.
    - Review your thinking with someone who knows more than you do.
    - Develop your clinical skills so that you can trust them. Examine the heart before looking at the echocardiogram report. When your diagnosis

consistently matches the report, your physical examination is reliable.

- You can develop clinical reasoning in the same way. Commit yourself to a differential diagnosis. When you consistently match the final diagnosis, your clinical reasoning is reliable.
- When you know that your skills in history taking, physical examination, and clinical reasoning are reliable, trust them. Say what you think. The correct diagnosis is *often* made by a junior team member, who may have given the case more thought or attention.
- Help out. There is an unwritten agreement that if you help others to do their work, they can use their freed time to teach you something.

PART II

ASSIMILATING INFORMATION

CHAPTER 11

Accessing the Medical Literature

Sources of Information

1. You will often find yourself in the predicament that you do not know, or do not recall, or only half recall, some piece of medical knowledge. Personal memory is indispensable, but fallible. Before you advise a patient, recommend a treatment, or record patient data, you need to be sure that what you're saying and doing is right.

   If you're not absolutely certain, check!

   Happily, there are numerous sources of information to help you educate yourself.
2. "**Expert Opinion.**" Others (e.g., other students, interns, residents, fellows, an attending, a nurse, a physician you meet in passing, a subspecialist) may know more than you do. You will often ask one of these people for information. This is helpful but not infallible. *If you're not absolutely certain, check!*

   Tip: Be wary of asking physicians to comment on a case in which they are not involved. A consultation is a formal mechanism by which a physician makes recommendations regarding a patient's care. The consultant performs a complete assessment and evaluation of the patient before rendering an opinion. It is unfair to grab a passing physician and ask him or her to render a meaningful opinion, except for simple points of fact. If you need help, consider a full consultation.

3. **Textbooks.** Textbooks are usually the best places to start your inquiry. They represent an overview that has usually synthesized the diverse opinions on a topic. They are not, however, completely up to date. Remember that a large text with a publication date of 1994 was probably printed in 1993 with chapters written in 1992.

   Textbooks also exist on computer. The most notable example is the *Scientific American Medicine* textbook, which is available on CD-ROM. Your medical center may provide such texts on a local computer network.

4. **References.** Specific references are available, as books and on computer, regarding many aspects of clinical medicine. These are described in Appendix 2.

5. **Journals.** Journal articles provide the most recent views on a given topic. However, they have several potential drawbacks. A journal article may reflect a partisan point of view. A journal article tends to magnify its own data and to minimize the significance of contradictory data. Finally, although it is tempting to quote the latest articles, the newest may not be the truest.

   Journals vary in their subject matter and the quality of their research. The better journals select articles by *peer review*, a process by which a group of specialists evaluate submitted materials. Journals that do not use peer review may not subject submitted articles to rigorous critique.

   There are several types of journal articles:

   - **Original Research**. The researcher formulates a hypothesis and gathers data to assess it.

- **Review.** The writer analyzes what has been written or said on a given topic. Variants are the editorial and the "point of view" article.
- **Meta-Analysis.** The author pools the data from several primary studies on the same topic. The advantages of doing so are that a large sample size is achieved, statistical associations are strengthened, and the effects of chance events that could occur at a single center are lessened. The disadvantages are that the different studies never have exactly the same population, intervention, outcome measures, or analysis, so that important distinctions can become blurred.
- **Consensus Recommendations.** An expert panel, usually under the auspices of a national organization such as the American College of Physicians or the National Institutes of Health, formulates a consensus view of a topic. These are intended to guide the physician in areas of controversy.
- **"Throwaways."** These journals are so named because they are delivered free to physicians. Articles in throwaways often provide practical guidelines not found in research articles, but quality varies widely. Most are not peer-reviewed.
- **Literature Review Journals.** Also called "literature surveillance journals," these journals provide critical analysis of current literature or issues. The best literary review journals are:
  - *Journal Watch*, published monthly by the Massachusetts Medical Society. Available by subscription ($55/yr for students and residents).
  - *ACP Journal Club*, published bimonthly by the American College of Physicians. Focuses on articles in internal medicine. Supplied free with subscriptions to the *Annals of Internal Medicine* ($42/yr for students; $59.25/yr for residents).
  - *The Medical Letter on Drugs and Therapeutics*,

published about three times a month by *The Medical Letter*, a nonprofit organization. Focuses on treatment issues, especially drug therapy. Available by subscription ($18.75/yr for students and residents). One of the great bargains in medical education.

The Computer Literature Search

1. ***Index Medicus.*** The *Index Medicus* is the full journal bibliography from the National Library of Medicine (NLM). The NLM is the largest medical library in the world. The *Index Medicus* is published monthly on paper and is accessed exactly like the index in a (gigantic) book. It contains only bibliographic information (not content) and is very unwieldy.
2. **MEDLINE** is the computer version of the *Index Medicus*. Articles are referenced according to author, title, "keywords," journal, date of publication, and medical subject headings.

   In addition to bibliographic information, abstracts of articles are also provided. These are invaluable for scanning the content of an article without physically finding it in the library. MEDLINE is published on CD-ROM. Articles appear about 1 month after publication.
3. There are several ways to access MEDLINE information. Your library may have the CD-ROM disks themselves. These are complete but expensive, so the library may have only one or two MEDLINE workstations. MEDLINE is not terribly user-friendly. However, several user-friendly software interfaces with the full MEDLINE database have been developed.

   Mini-MEDLINE presents MEDLINE data from an abridged journal list, comprising 300 to 500 journals (depending on date). Libraries often provide Mini-MEDLINE as part of their computerized card catalog. It is, however, rather slow and cumbersome.

Grateful Med® is a commercial software product for personal computers that provides a user-friendly interface, via modem, with MEDLINE. It is the most popular product of its type and can be purchased via advertisements in medical journals. Some physician's organizations offer *Grateful Med* at discounted prices.

Knowledge Finder® is an excellent MEDLINE interface for the MacIntosh computer, available on a local computer network or by CD-ROM. Other commercial products are available, including *BRS Colleague®*.

Professional reference librarians can perform searches for you (generally for a fee). The advantage of professional literature searching is completeness. The advantage of performing your own searches is that you can browse the fields of inquiry and get a sense of "what's out there."

4. How to search
   - Choose your topic. Medical topics have been catalogued into a list of terms called "medical subject headings" (MeSH). Thus, "colon cancer" fits under the MeSH topic, "colorectal neoplasms." Be patient. It takes a little practice and familiarity with the system to translate your formulation of topics into MeSH topics.
   - Choose the set of journals that you want to search. At minimum, you must select a time period; most programs can search 1 to 5 years at a time. Set your database according to the following:
     - **Time frame.** Usually begin with the most recent period, then move back as desired. Remember that the newest is not always the best.
     - **Completeness.** Most applications allow you to

choose between maximal completeness and maximal relevance.

- **Restrictions.** You can restrict your search to English language only, review articles only, humans only, etc.
- *Subheadings* allow you to hone in your search to a specific aspect of your topic such as treatment or epidemiology.
- **Boolean algebra.** To investigate a topic such as vitamin E in the prevention of CAD:
  - First search coronary artery disease ("A")
  - Then search Vitamin E ("B")
  - Then search "A" *AND* "B." This will provide all the articles that deal with both coronary artery disease and vitamin E.
  - Read the abstracts. Articles that seem pertinent to your needs can be tagged for subsequent saving or printing.
- Save or print your search. Searches can be downloaded to diskettes.

5. Tips for computer searches
   - Do them. Computer literature searches are the best way to access complete, up-to-date information.
   - Stay flexible; consider alternate formulations of search topics. In the vitamin E example, you may uncover important articles by searching the topic *myocardial infarction* in addition to *coronary artery disease.*
   - Some drugs are listed by the class of agent, rather than the drug name itself. For example, if you find no articles listed under the topic *terazosin,* try searching *alpha blockers.*
   - Remember that you have a lot of search options. If you find a useful article by a particular author, you can then search all the articles written by that author. If you half recall seeing an article in a particular journal, you can search all the articles ap-

pearing in that journal or all the articles on a given topic in a given journal.
- If you are having trouble finding pertinent articles, some software interfaces give you the option of searching according to free text, instead of MeSH headings only.

Critical Reading

1. Reading the medical literature presents two major problems. The first is volume; thousands of medical articles are published in hundreds of journals every year. It is impossible to read even the most important ones. The second problem is quality; many articles are deeply flawed in their design or analysis.
2. **The Problem of Volume.** Algorithms have been developed to evaluate articles while browsing, so that you can decide whether to read the article in depth. The most famous is the one designed at McMaster University, published in the *Canadian Medical Association Journal* in 1981.[1] In this algorithm, you screen for appropriate articles by addressing a short series of questions.
   - **Title.** Does it appear interesting and useful?
   - **Authors.** Do they have a reliable track record?
   - **Summary.** Would the results be useful, if they prove valid?
   - **Site.** Is it relevant to your practice site?
   - **Your Goals.** What are you trying to learn?
3. **The Problem of Quality.** Medical research is inherently imperfect. In medical experiments, the subjects are humans or other complex biologic phenomena. It is very difficult to assemble groups of people that differ only in a single variable. In addition, an intervention applied deliberately to human

[1]Department of Clinical Epidemiology and Biostatistics, McMaster University Health Sciences Centre. How to read clinical journals. Parts I–V. Can Med Assoc J Vol 124, 1981.

subjects must not be harmful to them; this limits the way in which many interventions can be studied.

The research and statistical techniques developed to compensate for these limitations can be quite complex. Nonetheless, a few guidelines for assessing the quality of a medical research article can help you to a reasoned evaluation. You must steer between two extremes: accepting every claim as true, on the one hand, and rejecting everything as fatally flawed, on the other.

4. **Study Designs.** These fit into two basic categories: descriptive and interventional.
5. **Descriptive Studies.** In these studies, the investigator describes a phenomenon. Descriptive studies fall into two main types.
   - **Case Report.** An interesting event, found in a relatively small number of patients, is described. These typically occur early in the recognition of a new syndrome, such as human Hantavirus infection.
   - **Prevalence Study.** The frequency of a finding in a given population is measured.
6. **Interventional Studies.** In these studies, the investigator observes the effects of an intervention on one group of subjects compared with another. The intervention could be determined by the investigator or by other circumstances. The four main types of interventional studies are listed here in order from strongest to weakest.
   - **Randomized Clinical Trial.** The study population is randomized either to receive or not to receive an intervention, and the subsequent outcome is measured. *Randomization* doesn't mean that the interventions occur "at random" or "by chance," but rather that a definite process is employed for assigning subjects randomly. The most common

process in current use is a computer-generated list of random numbers.

Example

> One thousand women with coronary artery disease are randomly assigned to receive vitamin E supplements or placebo; the rate of subsequent MI is then measured and compared in the two groups.

- **Cohort Study.** The study population either receives or does not receive an intervention, for wha tever reason, and the subsequent outcome is measured. The investigator does not control which subject receives which intervention.

Example

> In a group of 1000 women with coronary artery disease, 400 report taking vitamin E supplements and 600 do not. The rate of subsequent MI is then measured and compared in the two groups.

- **Case-Control Study.** The study population is divided into two groups: one that had experienced a certain outcome ("cases") and one that had not ("controls"). These groups are then studied for the presence or absence of a prior intervention or exposure.

Example

> In a group of 1000 women, 200 had had a prior MI and 800 had not. The women are questioned regarding their prior use of vitamin E supplements, and the rate of vitamin E use in the two groups is compared.

- **Case Series.** A study population with a certain

outcome is examined retrospectively for the presence of an intervention or exposure. There is no control group.

Example

> A group of 1000 women with MI is questioned regarding prior use of vitamin E supplements.

7. When evaluating journal articles, it is best to rely on a standard set of criteria. Some criteria apply to all articles.
   - Is the question under study clearly articulated?
   - Are the results, if *statistically* significant, also *clinically* significant? An article that demonstrates that a medication reduces BP by 1 mm Hg might have a *P* value of <.0001, but the finding is not clinically important.
   - Is the study design inherently strong?
   - When human subjects are involved is there a clear description of how the subjects were assembled and entered into the study?
   - Was the spectrum of patients broad enough to be applicable to other circumstances? Or to your clinical population?
   - Were satisfactory attempts made to eliminate, or to correct for, bias? *Bias* is the occurrence of systematic errors in collecting or interpreting data.[2]

     Selection bias occurs when patients are enrolled in a study, or subjected to an intervention, according to a variable that might be linked to the topic under study. For example, persons who choose to take vitamin supplements might also exercise more than those who do not.

     Recall bias occurs when persons are asked to remember prior health events, some of which may be more memorable than others. For exam-

---

[2]Hennekens, CH and Buring, JE: Epidemiology in Medicine. Boston, Little, Brown, 1987, p 4.

ple, persons with leukemia might be more likely to recall prior radiation exposure than others.

Interviewer bias occurs when investigators systematically solicit or elicit information differently in two different groups. For example, an investigator might ask persons with leukemia more emphatically about prior radiation exposure than other persons.

Two techniques used to correct for bias are:

- *Multivariate analysis*, in which a mathematical model seeks to factor in the relative weights of several variables on an outcome.
- *Stratification*, in which groups are divided into subgroups according to variables that might influence an outcome.

8. In addition, specific criteria for specific types of articles have been published.[3] These have been pioneered at McMaster University.

For Articles Relating to Diagnostic Tests

- Independent, blind comparison with a gold standard
- Adequate spectrum of patients: Severity, treated/untreated
- Clear description of referral pattern (patient collection)
- Clear description of the test (reproducible)
- Reproducible results among different observers
- Clear and sensible description of "normal"
- Contribution of the test to diagnosis, compared with other tests

For Articles Relating to Prognosis

- Inception cohort
- Clear description of referral pattern (patient collection)

[3]Sackett, DL, et al: Clinical Epidemiology: A Basic Science for Clinical Medicine. Boston, Little, Brown, 1991.

- Outcome criteria clinically important, objective, and "blind"
- Follow-up: Ideally complete; accept ≥80%
- Adjustment for extraneous prognostic factors

For Articles Relating to Etiology

- Unbiased assignment to intervention and measurement of outcome
- Clinical importance
- Consistency among diverse studies
- Correct temporal sequence between putative cause and effect
- Dose-response relationship (greater exposure leads to greater magnitude of outcome)

For Articles Relating to Treatment

- Random assignment of patients
- Outcome criteria clinically important, objective, and "blind"
- All outcome criteria reported
- Follow-up: Ideally complete; accept ≥80%
- Statistically *and clinically* significant
- Adverse effects reported
- Assessment of power for negative studies

For Review Articles

- Explicit criteria for selecting articles for review
- Assessment of the validity of the primary studies
- Analysis of differing results from the primary studies
- Appropriate combination of findings from the primary studies

For Meta-Analysis

- Explicit criteria for including and excluding studies
- Similar populations, interventions, and outcome measures among included studies

9. In discussing or presenting articles, it is best to follow a set format. I recommend the following se-

quence, which is modeled after that found in the *Annals of Internal Medicine*.

- Study objective
  What did the authors attempt to do?
- Study design
  Cohort study? Randomized clinical trial?
- Setting
  University health center ophthalmology clinic? Veteran's Administration hospital?
- Patients
  One thousand registered nurses responding to a questionnaire? All patients admitted to the coronary care unit for 6 months?
- Intervention
  What were the key variables distinguishing the study and the control groups?
- Main outcome measures
  What were the key issues being evaluated? Five-year mortality? Rate of improvement in a symptom score?
- Main results
  What values were obtained for the outcome measures?
- Conclusion
  What did the authors think they had shown?
- Your commentary
  What do you think they showed? How well does the article fulfill the criteria listed above?

Example

> *Reporting on an Article You Have Read*
>
> The study objective was to assess whether vitamin E supplementation reduces the risk of MI in women. The study was a cohort study. The setting was a large urban and suburban health maintenance organization. The patients consisted of 10,000 consecutively enrolled women, aged 40–65, who joined the HMO in 1985–6. The intervention was ingestion of vit-

amin E in doses ≥400 IU daily, as reported on a questionnaire completed at the time of enrollment. The main outcome measure was the occurrence of an MI as determined by review of billing submissions, during the period 1986–1995. The main results were as follows: of 2000 subjects who took vitamin E, 40 (2%) suffered MI. Of 8000 subjects who did not take vitamin E, 240 (3%) suffered MI. The relative risk of MI for subjects who took vitamin E was 0.67 ($P < .01$). The authors conclude that vitamin E supplementation reduces the risk of MI in women.

Comments: The study was fairly well designed. The inception cohort was well defined; however, there was no clear description of the referral pattern. While the outcome criterion of MI was clinically important, MIs may have been missed if the patient died abruptly and did not receive medical care, or if a bill was not submitted for some other reason. The follow-up was acceptable at 85%. There was no adjustment for other prognostic factors, such as smoking, exercise, hypertension, or family history; persons interested in taking vitamin E might also have chosen exercise and smoking cessation. There was no mention of side effects in the vitamin E group, and there was no attempt to assess whether the duration of vitamin E treatment correlated with the rate of MI. In sum, the article provides suggestive evidence that vitamin E may reduce the risk of MI in women, but it is too limited in study design to be conclusive.

CHAPTER 12

Interpreting Tests

General Principles

1. Tests might be ordered for several reasons:
   - *To evaluate suspected conditions.* You think that a person might have diabetes mellitus, and you order a serum glucose level.
   - *To screen for occult conditions.* You order a serum glucose level to detect otherwise unsuspected diabetes mellitus.
   - *"Routine."* You order the tests typically ordered for patients similar to yours.
   - *"To protect against accusations of omission."* You order a test so that no one can say you forgot to think of something. This occurs quite commonly, although it is more costly than useful.
2. The issue of routine blood tests has become quite controversial. Routine tests belong more to custom than to science. The advantage of routine admission testing is that it completes a standard database for all patients. Unsuspected conditions are identified, and a baseline for future comparison is established. One disadvantage of routine testing is its cost; the standard admission set that follows might cost $300 or more. With a few exceptions, it is unusual to detect an important but completely unsuspected disease based on routine blood testing alone. In the the example of PT/PTT analysis on basically healthy patients admitted for surgery, a hos-

pital that performs 1000 cholecystectomies a year might spend $42 × 1000 = $42,000 to detect one or two persons with unsuspected bleeding abnormalities.

An additional problem is the false positive. In testing for a condition with a low prevalence in the population under study, a positive test result is more likely to be a false positive than a true positive. Physicians, however, feel uncomfortable ascribing an abnormal result to a false positive without further testing. This means that every patient with an abnormal PT/PTT will have additional tests, causing further cost and delay.

There are few data to support the routine use of most of the tests routinely ordered. There are some data in favor of checking a CBC, glucose, and creatinine, for inpatients, and cholesterol, for outpatients. Children benefit from periodic lead screening.

3. The tests that are considered routine vary according to clinical setting and to individual practice or institutional styles.
   - **General Hospital Admission, Adult.** CBC, biochemistry panel, urinalysis, PT/PTT, chest x-ray, and electrocardiogram (EKG). Some hospitals include syphilis serology and the sedimentation rate.
   - **Psychiatric Admission.** Same as for the general hospital admission, plus thyroid tests and sometimes vitamin B_{12}.
   - **Surgical Admission.** Same as for the general hospital admission, plus a blood type and crossmatch.
   - **Pediatric Admission.** CBC, possibly chest x-ray.
   - **Outpatient Comprehensive Health Evaluation (Annual Physical).** CBC, biochemistry panel (with cholesterol), urinalysis, EKG for age ≥30 years.

- **Outpatient Obstetrics.** CBC, blood type and Rh factor, syphilis serology, rubella titre.
- **Nursing Home Admission.** CBC, biochemistry panel, urinalysis, chest x-ray, EKG, and tuberculosis skin testing.

For the intern and student, it is best to order whatever tests are routine for your situation. But stay tuned: the evidence supporting routine tests is scanty, and efforts to reduce costs may eliminate them.

4. **Guidelines for Ordering Tests.** For each test you are considering ordering, ask yourself the following:
   - *What information will be gained?*

     In a patient with acute, moderately severe back pain but no neurologic abnormalities, a spine magnetic resonance imaging (MRI) scan that shows a bulging disk may not mean a lot (although it will certainly cost a lot).
   - *How likely is the result to be abnormal?*

     If a diagnosis of acute intermittent porphyria is unlikely, spending $200 or so for the urine tests may not be warranted.
   - *Is the test painful or dangerous?*

     Even seemingly innocuous tests can be so.
   - *What does it cost?*

     Quite possibly, more than you think. An MRI scan of the knee cost some $1400 in New York in 1995. Prostate specific antigen cost $85 to $90.
   - *Has the test already been done?*

     It is not uncommon to see a patient with abnormal liver tests have the same hepatitis B serologies checked six different times.
   - *Would the result change the pretest probability significantly?*

     If the pretest probability is 60%, a test that when positive gives a posttest probability of 70%, and when negative 50%, should not be ordered (see Chapter 16).

- *Will the result have a consequence in action?*
  Will you do anything with the result? Or are you just satisfying your curiosity? Curiosity is a virtue, but it does not entitle you to a blank check for ordering tests.

Interpreting Blood Tests

Listed here is basic information for the common blood tests. Note that, while standard normal ranges are provided, these may vary from one laboratory to another. The units listed are those most commonly used in clinical practice. The differential diagnoses listed are highly condensed. Costs are for New York City, 1995.

Each test requires the right kind of sample. The glass tubes for blood collection are either empty or contain an additive that affects blood clotting. The type of tube is indicated by the color of its stopper.

1. Complete blood count (CBC)
   Description: Measures the number and size of cellular components of blood
   Technique: Coulter counter
   Sample: Plasma, 1 mL (purple-top tube)
   Cost: $15 to $26

   Components
   White blood cell (WBC) count
   Normal Range: 3.4 to 11.2 K/μL
   Elevated
   Reactive: Infection, trauma, surgery
   Primary: Leukemia
   Depressed
   Reactive: Chemotherapy, viral infections, overwhelming infections
   Primary: Bone marrow disease

   Red blood cell (RBC) count
   Normal Range: Male, 4.5 to 6.3 million/mL; female, 4.2 to 5.4 million/mL

Elevations and depressions should follow hemoglobin; disparities between RBC and hemoglobin reflect mean corpuscular volume (MCV)

Hemoglobin (Hgb)

Normal Range: Male, 14 to 18 g/dL; female, 12 to 16 g/dL

Elevated

Hemoconcentration: Volume depletion

Polycythemia: Essential or secondary

Depressed

Increased Destruction: Bleeding, hemolysis

Decreased Production: Substrate deficiency (iron, B_{12}), chronic disease, hematologic neoplasm

Hematocrit (Hct)

Normal Range: Male, 42 to 52 mL/dL; female, 37 to 47 mL/dL. (The units are also listed as "%," since the ratio of mL to dL is 1 : 100).

Elevations and depressions should follow Hgb; if not, disparities between RBC and hemoglobin reflect the patient's volume status.

Mean Corpuscular Volume (MCV)

Normal Range: 81 to 100 fL

Elevated

Megaloblastic anemia

Bone marrow infiltration or dysfunction

Liver Disease

Reticulocytosis

Some drugs

Depressed

Iron deficiency

Thalassemia trait

Lead poisoning

Sideroblastic anemias

Platelets (Plt)

Normal range: 150 to 450 K/μL

Elevated

Reactive marrow

Essential thrombocythemia

Depressed

Increased Destruction: Idiopathic thrombocytopenic purpura,. thrombotic thrombocytopenic purpura, disseminated intravascular coagulation

Decreased Production: Marrow suppression

Dilution (e.g., after blood transfusion)

Sequestration (splenomegaly)

2. Biochemistry Profile (Profile, SMA 20, SMA 26)

Description: Measures the concentrations of various salts, enzymes, and other substances in serum

Technique: Multichannel processor

Sample: Serum, 5 mL (red-top tube)

Cost: $31 to $58, depending on number of constituents

Components:

Sodium (Na)

Normal Range: 133 to 147 mmol/L

Elevated

Decreased water intake: Coma, decreased thirst

Increased water loss in urine, stool, skin, wounds, or respiratory tract

Sodium Loading: Iatrogenic, aldosterone effect

Depressed

Always evaluate volume status first!

Volume Depletion: Fluid loss from any cause

Volume Overload: Congestive heart failure, cirrhosis, nephrotic, edema

Euvolemia: Syndrome of inappropriate secretion of antidiuretic hormone (SIADH), Addison's disease, hypothyroidism

Potassium (K)

Normal Range: 3.2 to 5.2 mmol/L

Elevated

K Loading: Exogenous, cell lysis (rhabdomyolysis, tumor, etc.)

K Shift from Intracellular to Extracellular Compartment: Acidosis
K Retention: Renal failure, drug, renal tubular acidosis (type IV), low aldosterone
Spurious: Hemolysis in blood tube, leukocytosis

Depressed
Low intake (rare except iatrogenically)
K Shift from Extracellular to Intracellular Compartment: Alkalosis, insulin
K Loss: Renal (drug!), gastrointestinal (diarrhea, etc.), high aldosterone, renal tubular acidosis (type I and II)

Chloride (Cl)

Normal Range: 94 to 110 mmol/L

Generally follows sodium. Primary chloride disorders are unusual, except in the instances listed below.

Elevated
Chloride loading (especially "normal saline," a solution of sodium chloride)

Depressed
Nasogastric suctioning
Vomiting

Bicarbonate (HCO_3, CO_2)

Normal Range: 22 to 32 mmol/L

Elevated
Metabolic alkalosis (especially volume depletion)
Renal compensation for respiratory acidosis

Depressed
Metabolic acidosis (especially sepsis)
Renal compensation for respiratory alkalosis
Carbonic anhydrase inhibitors

Anion Gap (AG, "delta")

The anion gap is calculated: $AG = Na - (Cl + HCO_3)$. It represents the number of negatively charged ions that are not measured on the profile.

Normal Range: 5 to 15 mmol/L

Elevated

Metabolic acidosis from unmeasured anions:

Lactate (lactic acidosis, as in sepsis or unperfused tissue)

Acetoacetate (diabetic ketoacidosis, alcohol intoxication)

Methanol intoxication

Ethylene glycol intoxication

Salicylate intoxication

Depressed

Occasionally in multiple myeloma

Blood Urea Nitrogen (BUN)

Normal Range: 5 to 25 mg/dL

Elevated

Decreased renal function

Decreased renal perfusion

Blood in gastrointestinal tract

Depressed

Starvation

Catabolic illness

Creatinine (Cr)

Normal Range: 0.5 to 1.5 mg/dL

Elevated

Decreased renal function

Muscle breakdown

Depressed

Starvation

Catabolic illness

Blood Urea Nitrogen to Creatinine (BUN/Cr) Ratio

Normal Range: <20

Increased

Renal hypoperfusion (systemic volume depletion, systemic hypotension, congestive heart failure, cirrhosis, renal artery stenosis)

Depressed

Not significant

Serum Glutamic-Oxaloacetic Transaminase (SGOT), a.k.a. Aspartate Aminotransferase (AST)
Normal Range: 0 to 45 U/L
Elevated
Hepatocyte damage
Acute MI
Skeletal muscle damage
SGOT > SGPT often implies alcoholic hepatitis
Depressed
Not significant

Serum Glutamic-Pyruvic Transaminase (SGPT), a.k.a. Alanine Aminotransferase (ALT)
Normal Range: 0 to 45 U/L
Elevated
Hepatocyte damage
Acute MI
Skeletal muscle damage
Depressed
Not significant

Alkaline Phosphatase (Alk Phos)
Normal Range: 30 to 110 U/L
Elevated
Hepatobiliary disease (cholestasis, biliary obstruction)
"Interstitial" liver process
Bone disease: Paget's disease, metastases, hyperparathyroidism
Placental production: pregnancy, especially with complications
Depressed
Not significant

γ-glutamyltransferase (GGT)
The main function of GGT is to assess the source of an elevated alk phos. If alk phos is elevated, an elevated GGT indicates a hepatobiliary source. Normal GGT indicates a bone or placental

source. An alternative enzyme that plays the same role is *5′-nucleotidase.*

Normal Range: 9 to 55 U/L

Elevated

Hepatobiliary disease

Acute pancreatitis

Depressed

Not significant

Bilirubin (Bili)

Normal Range: 0.1 to 1.0 mg/dL

Bilirubin should be considered in terms of its two components:

Direct Bilirubin (Direct Bili)

Normal Range: 0.1 to 0.4 mg/dL

Elevated: Biliary obstruction, cholestasis, hepatocyte dysfunction

Depressed: Not significant

Indirect bilirubin (Indirect Bili)

Normal Range: 0.1 to 0.8 mg/dL

Elevated: Hepatocyte dysfunction, decreased hepatic conjugation, hemolysis

Depressed: Not significant

Albumin (Alb)

Normal Range: 3 to 5 g/dL

Elevated

Volume depletion

Depressed

Catabolic states (starvation, cancer, chronic infections, chronic inflammatory disease)

Protein loss (nephrotic syndrome, burn, protein-losing enteropathy)

Globulin (Glob)

Normal Range: 1.8 to 3.3 g/dL

Elevated

Immune activation (infection, collagen-vascular diseases)

Primary hematologic disorder: Myeloma, Waldenström's macroglobulinemia

Depressed

Not significant

Protein (Pro)

Pro = sum of albumin and globulin; analyze them independently.

Normal Range: 5.5 to 8.0 g/dL.

Lactate Dehydrogenase (LDH)

Normal Range: 80 to 225 U/L

Elevated

Any cell breakdown, especially acute MI, hemolysis, liver disease, lymphoma

Pneumocystis pneumonia

Depressed

Not significant

Creatine Phosphokinase, Creatine Kinase (CPK, CK)

Normal Range: 0 to 225 U/L

Elevated

Any form of muscle damage: MI, rhabdomyolysis, intramuscular injection, trauma

Isoenzymes are useful in diagnosis of acute MI (MB fraction >5%).

Depressed

Not significant

Calcium (Ca)

Normal Range: 8.5 to 10.5 mg/dL

If the serum albumin is low, calcium should be adjusted; Ca decreases 0.8 mg/dL for every decrease 1.0 mg/dL alb. For example, if Ca is 8.0 with alb 3.0, "corrected Ca" is 8.8.

Elevated

Hyperparathyroidism

Malignancy

Vitamin D intoxication

Thiazides
Granulomatous diseases

Depressed

Hypoparathyroidism
Renal failure
Low vitamin D
Transfusion

Phosphorus (PO_4, Phos)

Normal Range: 2.2 to 4.2 mg/dL

Elevated

Hypoparathyroid, renal failure, cell lysis

Depressed

Hyperparathyroid, starvation

Cholesterol (Chol)

It is better to think of desired ranges rather than normal values, since the usual values of cholesterol in Americans lead to heart disease.

"Desired" range: Less than 200 mg/dL

Elevated

Lipid disorders
Obesity
Thyroid disease

Depressed

Catabolic processes
Cancer
HIV infection

Cholesterol values are most meaningful when total cholesterol, high-density lipoprotein (HDL), low-density lipoprotein (LDL), and triglycerides (TG) are considered together.

Convenient rule of thumb: $LDL < TC - HDL - \frac{TG}{5}$

Interpreting Chest X-rays

1. Nearly every patient receives a chest x-ray on hospital admission and during the evaluation of a host

of clinical problems. It is essential that you know how to read a chest x-ray.

2. Chest x-rays can be performed by a number of techniques.
   - **Posterior-anterior (PA) and lateral.** With the patient standing, two views are obtained: 1) back to front and 2) right side to left. This technique gives the best quality films.
   - **Anterior-posterior (AP) sitting or supine.** With the patient sitting or lying down, one view is obtained, front to back. AP films are obtained when the patient is unable to stand. Their quality is inferior to PA/lateral films; in particular, the heart size is magnified.
   - **Portable Films.** These films are obtained when a patient is too unstable for transport to the Radiology Department. Portable films are always AP sitting or supine, and their quality is inferior to films obtained in the Radiology Department.
   - **Lateral Decubitus Films.** These films are taken with the patient lying on the side and are useful in assessing pleural effusions.
   - **Apical Lordotic Films.** These films are taken with the patient leaning forward and are useful for evaluating the lung apices or a suspected pulmonary nodule.
3. You will be more effective when reading chest x-rays if you develop a protocol for looking at films. By sticking to a sequence, you will look carefully at each aspect of the film and avoid overlooking important areas. Note that there are four main foci of attention in each of the six categories described here.
   - **Bones**
     - Spine
     - Shoulder
     - Ribs
     - Sternum (on lateral)

- **Soft tissues**
  - Breasts
  - Axillae
  - Thyroid (enlarged?)
  - Diaphragms
- **Mediastinum**
  - Airway deviation or narrowing
  - Great vessels
  - Mass
  - Hila
- **Heart**
  - Heart size
  - Chamber enlargement
  - Pericardium (effusion?)
  - Valves
- **Thoracic cavity**
  - Pleural effusion?
  - Pleural mass
  - Pneumothorax
  - Calcifications
- **Lung**
  - Degree of aeration
  - Blood vessels
  - Interstitium
  - Parenchyma

4. Cardinal findings on chest x-ray
   - **Infiltrate.** Infiltrates are irregular densities in the lung fields. They fall into two main patterns: alveolar and interstitial. *Alveolar infiltrates* are irregular, confluent opacities caused by filling of the alveoli with fluid or cells, as occurs in pneumonia, pulmonary edema, or alveolar cell carcinoma. They may be convex or streaky, but they follow the lobar anatomy of the lung. *Interstitial infiltrates* are linear opacities that follow the interstitium. They are caused by interstitial pneumonias, such as *Pneumocystis*; interstitial edema, as in congestive heart failure; interstitial spread of neoplasm; and interstitial lung disease.

- **Nodule.** A nodule is a circumscribed, usually convex opacity in the lung. A large nodule is called a "mass." Common causes include lung cancer, metastatic carcinoma, granuloma, and fungal disease. Calcifications usually imply an old granuloma. *Cavitation*, an area of central clearing, is common in tuberculosis and lung abscesses.
- **Pleural Effusion.** A *pleural effusion* is a collection of fluid in the pleural space. When small, it may cause only blunting of the costophrenic angles, especially on the lateral view. When large, it causes a solid density in the inferior thoracic cavity with a curved top surface; occasionally, the effusion can cause opacity of the entire hemithorax. When a pleural effusion is suspected, the logical next step is to perform a lateral decubitus film. (Free fluid layers on the dependent side.)
- **Pneumothorax.** A *pneumothorax* is a collection of air in the pleural space. It appears as an area of decreased density at the margin of the lung field; crowding of vessels in the remaining lung often occurs. When under positive pressure, it is called a *tension pneumothorax* and causes shift of the mediastinum to the opposite side. When not under pressure, it may cause mediastinal shift to the same side.
- **Pleural Mass.** A *pleural mass* appears as a rounded projection from the chest wall. The paradigmatic cause is mesothelioma.
- **Cardiomegaly.** The normal heart (in adults) is $\leq\frac{1}{2}$ the chest width on a PA projection. The heart may be diffusely enlarged in patients with dilated cardiomyopathy or congestive heart failure. *Pericardial effusion* can cause a similar appearance but more commonly looks like a centrally located water balloon.
- **Chamber Enlargement.** *Left ventricular enlargement* causes a "boot-shaped" appearance with displacement down and posterior. *Left atrial enlarge-*

ment causes a bulging left atrial appendage, a double density over the mediastinum, an elevated left mainstem bronchus, and (on the lateral) a posterior displacement of the esophagus. *Right ventricular enlargement* causes increased prominence of the lower right heart border, elevation of the left ventricular apex, and (on the lateral) filling of the retrosternal space. *Right atrial enlargement* causes bulging of the right heart border.

5. Additional tips for interpreting chest x-rays
   - In a woman, make sure both breasts are present.
   - An opacity in the area of the upper sternum may be a submanubrial goiter.
   - Always check to see if air is present under the diaphragm. This indicates perforation of an abdominal viscus, a medical emergency. It is also found after deliberate entry into the abdominal cavity, as in surgery, laparoscopy, paracentesis, and hysterosalpingography.
   - A bubbly, spongy appearance to the soft tissues indicates subcutaneous emphysema, the entry of air into the skin and underlying fat. This can occur after pneumothorax.
   - If the heart is diffusely enlarged but the pulmonary vessels are not widened, think of pericardial effusion.
   - *Congestive heart failure* progresses on chest x-rays in stages.
     - **Pulmonary Vascular Congestion.** Blood vessels to the upper lungs are selectively dilated.
     - **Interstitial Edema.** *Kerley B lines* (short horizontal lines in the lateral lower lung fields) are evident.
     - **Alveolar Edema.** The alveoli fill with fluid and are seen as fluffy opacities, first in the perihilar region and then throughout the lungs. Remember that alveolar edema can also occur in non-

cardiogenic pulmonary edema, such as adult respiratory distress syndrome (ARDS).

Interpreting Electrocardiograms

1. Most patients age 30 or older, whether inpatients or outpatients, will have an EKG. In EKG interpretation, it is easy to immerse yourself in detail or obscurity while missing the big picture. As in many areas of clinical medicine, following a set protocol will keep you on course.

The protocol for EKG interpretation is as follows:
Rate
Rhythm
Intervals (PR, QRS, QT, QT_c)
Axis
P-wave morphology
QRS morphology
ST-segment morphology
T-wave morphology

2. **Rate.** Rate is measured in beats per minute. At the standard paper speed on an EKG machine, each small box horizontally is equal to 0.04 second. Each large box consists of five small boxes and thus equals 0.20 second. Five large boxes equal 1 second.

   The simplest way to measure rate is to count the number of big boxes between consecutive QRS complexes. If QRS complexes occur at every big box, they are occurring 0.2 second apart. Five occur in 1 second, and 300 in 60 seconds. Thus, the heart rate (HR) is 300 bpm. Similarly, if QRS complexes occur at every other big box, they are occurring every 0.4 second, and the HR is $60 \div 0.4 = 150$. You can continue this process, or you can refer to the following table.

Number of Big Boxes Between QRS Complexes	Heart Rate (bpm)
1	300
2	150
3	100
4	75
5	60
6	50

If there are more than six big boxes between consecutive QRS complexes, count the number between two QRS intervals and divide the rate by two.

The normal HR is 60 to 100 bpm. A HR 42 to 60 bpm is not uncommon in trained athletes but may be abnormal in others.

3. **Rhythm.** First, look for the P wave, then for the relation between the P wave and the QRS complex. The main rhythms are as follows:
   - **Normal Sinus Rhythm.** Every P wave has normal morphology and is followed by a QRS complex. The PR interval is constant and ranges from 0.12 second (three small boxes) to 0.20 second (five small boxes).
   - **Atopic Atrial Rhythm.** The P wave does not arise in the sinoatrial node and has an abnormal morphology. However, it is followed by a QRS complex with an appropriate interval.
   - **Junctional Rhythm.** Either no P wave is visible or it is inverted and follows the initial part of the QRS complex. The QRS complex is normal.
   - **Supraventricular Tachycardia.** No P wave is visible. The HR is >100 bpm and typically is in the range of 240 bpm. The QRS complexes are narrow and regular.
   - **Atrial Fibrillation.** No P wave is visible. The HR is typically rapid but may be normal. The QRS

complexes are narrow but irregular, without any pattern evident.

- **Atrial Flutter.** P waves occur at a very rapid rate, typically 200 to 300 bpm, and assume a sawtooth pattern. QRS complexes are narrow and occur at integer multiples of the P wave (e.g., every third or every fourth P wave.)
- **Idioventricular Rhythm.** Either no P wave is visible or it is inverted and follows the initial part of the QRS complex. The HR is 40 to 100 bpm, usually at the lower end. The QRS complex is widened but regular.
- **Ventricular Tachycardia.** Either no P wave is visible or it is inverted and follows the initial part of the QRS complex. The HR is >100 bpm. The QRS complex is widened but regular.
- **Ventricular Fibrillation.** No P wave is visible. QRS complexes are wide and irregular, without an apparent pattern.

4. **Intervals.** There are three important intervals:
   - **PR Interval.** The PR interval is the span between the beginning of the P wave and the beginning of the QRS complex. The normal PR interval is 0.12 to 0.20 second.

     PR <0.12 second indicates preexcitation, as can occur in the Wolff-Parkinson-White syndrome or an ectopic atrial rhythm.

     PR >0.20 second indicates heart block:
     - **First-Degree Heart Block.** PR >0.20 second; PR otherwise normal.
     - **Second-Degree Heart Block, Type I (Wenckebach).** The PR intervals progressively increase until one P wave is not followed by a QRS; the cycle then resumes.
     - **Second-Degree Heart Block, Type II.** The PR intervals remain constant, but, at regular intervals, a QRS complex fails to occur.
     - **Third-Degree Heart Block.** Both P waves and QRS complexes occur at regular intervals, but

   there is no relation between the P waves and the QRS complexes.

- **QRS Interval.** The QRS interval is the span between the beginning of the QRS complex and the beginning of the ST segment. The normal QRS interval is ≤0.12 second (three small boxes).

  QRS >0.12 second can occur in:
  - Junctional or ventricular rhythms
  - Aberrant conduction between the atrium and ventricle
- **QT Interval.** The QT interval is the span between the beginning of the QRS complex and the end of the T wave. Because the QT interval varies with HR, one usually speaks of the corrected QT interval, QT_c. QT_c can be calculated as $QT_c = QT/\sqrt{RR}$. The normal QT_c interval is ≤0.4 second (two big boxes).

5. **Axis.** Although all EKG waves have axes, the most important axis is the QRS axis. The QRS axis can easily be calculated by comparing the magnitude and direction of the QRS complexes in leads I and aVL; it is the direction of the vector sum of these complexes. Thus, if the QRS is tall in I and flat in aVL, the axis is 0°. If the QRS is flat in I and tall in aVL, the axis is 90°. If the QRS has equal magnitude in I and aVL, the axis is 45°. If the QRS is twice as tall in I as in aVL, the axis is 30°. And so on. Axis calculation takes some practice; you should consult an EKG text if it is unclear.

   The interpretation of the QRS axis is as follows:
   - Axis 0° to 90°: Normal axis
   - Axis −90° to 0°: Left-axis deviation
   - Axis 90° to 180°: Right-axis deviation
6. **P-wave morphology.** The normal P wave is upright in leads I and aVL, with a height of ≤3 mm, and is smoothly contoured. Forms of abnormal P waves include:

- **Inverted P Waves.** These indicate either an ectopic atrial rhythm or retrograde conduction from the ventricle to the atrium.
- **Tall P Waves.** These indicate atrial enlargement. P-wave enlargement in leads I and II indicates left atrial enlargement, especially if the P wave is notched. P-wave enlargement in leads II, III, and aVF indicates right atrial enlargement, especially if the P wave is peaked.
- **Biphasic P Waves.** A P wave with a positive and then a negative deflection is normal in V_1. If the negative deflection is significantly larger than the positive, or if a biphasic pattern occurs in V_2, this is another sign of left atrial enlargement.

7. **QRS Morphology.** A Q wave is normal in leads III and aVR. A small Q wave (≤2 mm) can be normal in leads I, aVL, aVF, V_5, and V_6. *Any other Q waves are abnormal* and are likely to indicate either previous MI or aberrant conduction.

   The normal QRS amplitude varies from one lead to another.

   - *Low QRS amplitude* (<5 mm in all limb leads) is abnormal and implies pericardial effusion or heart failure.
   - *High QRS amplitude* is defined differently by different authorities. In the simplest version, one adds the amplitude in V_1 to the R amplitude in V_5 or V_6 (whichever is taller). If this sum is ≥35 mm, *left ventricular hypertrophy* is present. If the R wave in V_1 is taller than the S wave, *right ventricular hypertrophy* is present.
   - *Bundle branch block* occurs when one of the fascicles in the intraventricular septum fails to conduct properly. It is therefore often called "fascicular block." If the fascicle to the left ventricle malfunctions, *left bundle branch block* appears as a widened QRS complex that is strongly negative in V_1 and strongly positive in V_6. If the fas-

cicle to the right ventricle malfunctions, *right bundle branch block* appears as a widened QRS complex that is strongly positive in V_1 and strongly negative in V_6.

Bundle branch blocks are especially important because they interfere with the interpretation of the QRS complex. If bundle branch block is present, Q waves cannot be interpreted to mean a myocardial infarction; ST changes cannot be interpreted to mean ischemia; and QRS prolongation cannot be interpreted to mean a junctional or ventricular rhythm.

8. **ST-Segment Morphology.** The normal ST segment is isoelectric. *ST elevation* occurs in acute MI. Other patterns of ST elevation can occur in acute pericarditis and as a normal variant. *ST depression* occurs in myocardial ischemia without infarction.
9. **T-Wave Morphology.** The normal T wave is upright in leads I, II, and V_1 to V_4. The height is <5 mm in the limb leads and <10 mm in the precordial leads. Forms of abnormal T waves include:
   - *T-wave inversion*, which occurs in myocardial ischemia
   - *Tall, peaked T waves*, which occur in hyperkalemia and myocardial ischemia
10. Cardinal findings on EKG
    - *Myocardial infarction*
      - ST elevation.
      - T-wave inversion.
      - Peaked T waves.
      - Loss of previously existing R waves.
      - Q waves generally occur 24 to 72 hours after the infarction but can occur earlier.
    - *Myocardial ischemia without infarction* (angina)
      - ST depression
      - T-wave inversion
      - Peaked T waves
    - *Acute pericarditis*

- ST elevation in most or all leads

11. Additional tips for interpreting EKGs
    - The first six leads are called the "limb leads": I, II, III, aVR, aVL, and aVF. The other six leads are called the precordial leads: V_1 to V_6.
    - Leads are associated, not entirely accurately, with anatomic regions of the left ventricle.
        - Leads I and aVL are associated with the lateral wall.
        - Leads II, III, and aVF are associated with the inferior wall.
        - Leads V_1 and V_2 are associated with the anteroseptal region.
        - Leads V_3 and V_4 are associated with the anterior wall.
        - Leads V_5 and V_6 are associated with the anterolateral wall.
    - EKG changes that occur in an anatomic distribution are much more significant than those that do not.
    - **J-point Elevation.** Many normal persons, especially young African-American men, will have ST elevation in the precordial leads. This can look different from the ST elevation accompanying acute MI in that the ST segment makes an acute angle with the end of the QRS complex.
    - If an EKG isn't making any sense, consider retaking the tracing with careful attention to placement of the leads. Misplaced leads can throw everything off.

CHAPTER 13

Approaches to Common Clinical Problems

Clinicians are problem solvers. Although there are hundreds of clinical problems that might present in the course of time, the common problems occur almost every day. This chapter provides a practical method for approaching 10 of the most common inpatient problems and five of the most common outpatient problems.

The issue of clinical problem solving is developed at length in Part III. For the present purposes, a clinical problem is approached as follows:

1. Definition of the problem
2. Differential diagnosis
3. Management: focused history, focused physical examination, focused laboratory tests, treatment

Focused means that the investigation concentrates on the issues at hand. If the patient has acute dyspnea, you do not need to examine for a succussion splash or for dysdiadokinesia.

The problems analyzed here are listed in the clinical order,* familiar from the physical examination, that

---

*This order was first described on an Egyptian papyrus dating from about 1600 BC.

begins with vital signs and proceeds through the organ systems, cephalad to caudal (head to tail).

Inpatient Problems	Outpatient Problems
Hypotension	Fatigue
Fever	Hypertension
Tachycardia	Cough
Pain	Joint pain
Chest pain	Rash
Dyspnea	
Abdominal pain	
Acute renal failure	
Altered mental status	
Anemia	

Inpatient Problems

Hypotension

DEFINITION

Hypotension is defined as arterial BP inadequate to perfuse tissues. This threshold will vary somewhat from person to person. Tissue hypoperfusion usually occurs for mean BP <80 mm Hg, or for systolic BP <90 mm Hg.

DIFFERENTIAL DIAGNOSIS

Since normal BP requires blood, vascular tone, and a pumping heart, hypotension occurs when any one of these components fails.

1. Inadequate volume
   - Volume depletion
   - Hemorrhage
   - "Third spacing"
2. Inadequate vascular tone
   - Sepsis
   - Adrenal insufficiency
   - Anaphylaxis

- Vasodilator therapy

3. Inadequate cardiac function
   - MI
   - Cardiac arrhythmia
   - Severe valvular disease
   - Congestive heart failure
   - Cardiac tamponade

MANAGEMENT

1. **Assessment of Severity.** If the patient is not mentating clearly, critical hypotension is present.
   - Signal for cardiac arrest (Code Blue, Code 9). This will mobilize a team specifically designated for this emergency.
   - Place the patient in Trendelenburg position (head downward).
   - Administer intravenous fluids.
   - Then proceed to the next step.

   If the patient is mentating clearly, proceed to the next step.
2. Focused history
   - Evidence of volume loss: Diuretics, diarrhea, burns; oliguria
   - Evidence of hemorrhage: Bleeding, trauma
   - Evidence of infection: Fever, cough, dysuria
   - Evidence of adrenal insufficiency: Glucocorticoid therapy, hypopituitary syndrome
   - Evidence of anaphylaxis or vasodilation: Recent drug administration
   - Evidence of MI: Chest pain
   - Evidence of arrhythmia: Palpitations
   - Prior valvular disease
   - Evidence of tamponade: Malignancy, chest trauma
3. Focused physical examination
   - **Heart Rate.** If the HR is not increased (>100) in the setting of hypotension, either primary bradycardia or a heart-slowing drug is present.

     If the HR is irregular, the patient has an arrhythmia that may be contributing to hypotension

- **Orthostatic Blood Pressure.** A drop of ≥15 mm Hg in BP, or an increase of ≥10 bpm in HR, indicates inadequate volume or vasodilatation.
- Evidence of hemorrhage: Stool guaiac testing, asymmetric pulses, flank hematoma.
- Evidence of vasodilation: The normal response to hypotension is arterial vasoconstriction, which leaves the extremities cool and pale. If they are warm or flushed, inappropriate vasodilatation is present and is the likely cause of hypotension.
- Evidence of glucocorticoid therapy: Cushingoid facies, striae.
- Evidence of anaphylaxis: Edema, wheezes, stridor.
- Evidence of MI: S_4 gallop.
- Evidence of severe valvular disease: Murmur, cardiomegaly.
- Evidence of congestive heart failure: Jugular venous distention, rales, cardiomegaly, S_3 gallop, peripheral edema.
- Evidence of tamponade: Pulsus paradoxicus, jugular venous distention.

4. Focused diagnostic testing
   - CBC
   - EKG
   - Consider: chest x-ray, arterial blood gas, electrolytes
5. Treatment
   - Administer intravenous fluids.
   - Position patient in supine or Trendelenburg position.
   - If orthostatic hypotension and peripheral vasoconstriction are present, the patient has inadequate intravascular volume. Emphasize fluid administration, and search for sources of fluid loss.

Give special attention to the possibility of hemorrhage.

- If orthostatic hypotension and peripheral vasodilatation are present, the patient has inadequate vascular tone. Administer fluids and consider treatment for causes of vasodilatation with antibiotics (for sepsis), glucocorticoids (for adrenal insufficiency), epinephrine (for anaphylaxis), or vasoconstrictors.
- If orthostatic hypotension is not present, the patient has inadequate cardiac function. If the EKG demonstrates myocardial ischemia, treat with oxygen; with nitrates, beta blockers, or calcium channel blockers (if tolerated by BP); with heparin; or with thrombolytic agents. If arrhythmia is present, treat for same. If signs of tamponade are present, consider pericardiocentesis.

Fever

DEFINITION

Fever is defined as an elevation of body temperature. Normal body temperature varies more than is commonly thought and usually reaches daily maximum at about 4 PM. The range defined as normal varies according to the site of measurement. Fever is usually said to be present if the temperature is ≥38°C for oral temperatures or ≥38.5°C for rectal, core, or tympanic temperatures.

DIFFERENTIAL DIAGNOSIS

1. Infection
2. Systemic inflammatory states
   - Collagen-vascular disorders
   - Vasculitis
   - Lymphoproliferative disorders

3. Focal inflammatory states
   - Pericarditis
   - Acute MI
   - Pulmonary embolism
   - Hepatitis (autoimmune, alcoholic)
   - Acute cholecystitis
   - Pancreatitis
   - Whipple's disease
   - Inflammatory bowel disease
   - Deep vein thrombosis
   - Other tissue infarction
4. Allergy
   - Drug reaction
   - Allergic pneumonitis
5. Neoplasm
   - Lymphoma
   - Leukemia
   - Carcinoma: Kidney, liver, esophagus, stomach
   - Melanoma
   - Hepatic metastases
   - Atrial myxoma
6. Hypothalamic dysfunction
   - Hypothalamic stroke or trauma
   - Neuroleptic malignant syndrome
   - Malignant hyperthermia syndrome
7. Atelectasis? (reported to be a cause of postoperative fever)
8. Increased environmental temperature (heatstroke)

MANAGEMENT

1. Focused history
   - Time course
   - Localizing symptoms
   - Medication use
   - Travel
   - Night sweats?
   - Rigor?

2. Focused physical examination
   - Vital signs
   - Localized findings
   - Lymphadenopathy
   - Signs of deep vein thrombosis
   - Inflammation at catheter sites
   - Skin: Wounds, decubiti, rash
3. Focused diagnostic tests
   - CBC
   - Urinalysis
   - Chest x-ray
   - Consider: Liver function tests, blood cultures, sedimentation rate
4. Treatment
   - Some severe types of infection, if they are even suspected, should be treated immediately, after diagnostic tests have been conducted. These infections include sepsis, bacterial meningitis, bacteremia in neutropenic hosts, or cellulitis with gas-forming organisms.
   - If a significant infection is suspected, antibiotics should often be started empirically, after appropriate diagnostic tests have been performed. *Empiric treatment* means that, although the causative organism has not been identified conclusively, the possible causative organisms have been considered. Antibiotics are chosen to cover this group of possible etiologic agents. For example, in a patient with cellulitis, an antibiotic that covers Streptococcus and Staphylococcus species is chosen.
   - If no infectious syndrome is identified, and if the patient does not appear severely ill, it is often best to perform appropriate diagnostic tests and then to wait for their results before starting empiric therapy.
   - Temperature >40°C orally is dangerous and should be reduced by antipyretics, cold compresses, alcohol baths, cooling blanket, or (in extreme cases) immersion.

TIPS: CAUSES OF FEVER

The *most common sites of infection in hospitalized patients* are:

- The lung: Pneumonia
- The urinary tract: Cystitis, pyelonephritis
- The skin: Wounds, cellulitis, catheter infection, and decubitus ulcer

These have been immortalized as "wind, water, and wound."

The *most common causes of noninfectious fever in hospitalized patients* are:

- Drug reaction
- Deep vein thrombosis
- Pulmonary embolism

The *most common causes of fever in ambulatory patients* are:

- Viral syndromes
- Respiratory infections
- Urinary tract infections
- Cellulitis

The *most common causes of sustained fever in hospitalized patients* are:

- Endocarditis
- Osteomyelitis
- Hepatitis
- Drug fever
- Malignancy

The syndrome of *fever of unknown origin* (FUO) consists of a pattern of sustained fever with negative diagnostic tests. Common causes include:

- Endocarditis with fastidious organisms (those that are difficult to culture)
- Drug fever
- Tuberculosis
- Neoplasm

- Abscess
- Osteomyelitis
- Collagen-vascular disorders and vasculitis

Common causes of fever in patients with HIV infection are:

- Viral infections: Cytomegalovirus, Epstein-Barr virus, herpes simplex virus, HIV itself
- Bacterial infections: Pneumonia, syphilis, salmonella
- Mycobacterial infections: Tuberculosis, mycobacteria avium complex
- Fungal infections: Histoplasmosis, toxoplasmosis, candidiasis, coccidiomycosis
- Protozoal infections: Pneumocystis, amebiasis
- Neoplasm, especially lymphoma
- Drug reaction

In a hospitalized patient with fever, if the cause is not apparent by the history and examination, a minimal work-up includes CBC, chest x-ray, urinalysis, and blood cultures. Two sets of blood cultures are required; they should be drawn from 2 different sites, at least 30 minutes apart.

High fevers with rigors imply bacterial infections, often with bacteremia. Any patient with a shaking chill should have blood cultures performed.

Extreme temperature elevation (≥41°C orally) is uncommon and should make you think of noninfectious causes of fever, especially the hypothalamic, neoplastic, and environmental processes described previously.

TIPS: FEVER AFTER SURGERY

Fever is common after surgery and may not indicate infection. The cause of noninfectious postoperative fever is unknown but may involve the release of tissue pyrogens or pulmonary atelectasis. Fever may be low or intermediate (38°C to 39°C orally) during the first

24 hours after surgery and should then decrease each day. Higher fevers, shaking chills, prolonged or rising fevers, or profuse sweating imply infection or thrombosis.

All patients who develop fever after surgery should be evaluated. If the fever is low-grade, the patient appears well, and the history and physical exam are unremarkable, no further workup is immediately necessary. Otherwise, the diagnostic tests discussed previously should be performed.

Common infections after surgery include:

- Aspiration pneumonia
- Catheter-related urinary tract infections
- Catheter-related infections of the skin, vessel, or bloodstream
- Wound infection
- Abscess

Other common causes of postsurgical fever include:

- Deep vein thrombosis
- Drug fever

TIPS: TREATMENT OF FEVER

Antipyretics, such as acetaminophen, may be given *after* a fever has occurred *and has been evaluated.* Antipyretics given under other conditions may mask fever and obscure a crucial vital sign. Avoid ordering antipyretics PRN or around the clock; if a patient has a fever, you want to know about it.

Even when an infection is being properly treated, fevers may take several days to resolve. The sign of an infection responding to treatment is a progressive decrease in the daily maximum temperature, *Tmax*. A patient with pyelonephritis will typically begin with a temperature of 39.5°C orally; a typical response to appropriate antibiotics would mean a Tmax of 39.0°C on day 1, 38.5°C on day 2, 38.0°C on day 3, and then no further fever. A deviation from this pattern may indicate that the infection is not being adequately treated.

Closed-space infections, such as abscesses, cannot in general be cured with antibiotics alone. They should be drained.

Infections involving synthetic materials, such as vascular or urinary catheters, prosthetic cardiac valves, vascular grafts, and artificial joints, often require that the material be removed.

In choosing antibiotics, try to find the agent with the narrowest spectrum that covers the likely causative organisms. Using an antibiotic with an unnecessarily broad spectrum of activity promotes the development of resistant organisms, increases the cost of treatment, and predisposes to side effects.

Tachycardia

DEFINITION

Tachycardia is defined as HR >100. Note that an HR of 80 to 100 bpm is unusual for healthy young persons and may be inappropriately rapid.

DIFFERENTIAL DIAGNOSIS

1. Sinus tachycardia
   - Hypotension
   - Inadequate intravascular volume
   - Fever
   - Increased catecholamine states: Fear, anxiety, pain, stress
   - Hyperthyroidism
   - Anemia
   - Exercise
   - From medications: Theophylline, sympathomimetics, vasodilators
2. Ventricular arrhythmias
   - Ventricular tachycardia (VTach)
   - Ventricular fibrillation (VFib)
3. Supraventricular arrhythmias

- Supraventricular tachycardia (SVT)
- Atrial fibrillation (AFib)

MANAGEMENT

1. Focused history
   - Evidence of systemic hypotension: Lightheadedness
   - Evidence of inadequate volume: Oliguria
   - History of fever
   - Evidence of fear, pain, exercise, etc.
   - Evidence of hyperthyroidism: Weight loss, heat intolerance, diarrhea
   - History of recent medication
2. Focused physical examination
   - Blood pressure with orthostatic maneuver
   - Evidence of vasoconstriction: Cool or pale extremities
   - Temperature
   - Evidence of hyperthyroidism: Increased reflexes, tremor, goiter, proptosis
   - Evidence of anemia: Pallor
   - Evidence of arrhythmia: Peripheral and apical pulses
3. Focused diagnostic testing
   - EKG
   - Consider: CBC, thyroid tests
4. Treatment
   - If sinus tachycardia is present on EKG, identify the underlying cause as outlined previously.
   - If a cardiac arrhythmia is present on EKG, treat for same:

     VTach: Lidocaine, procainamide, or cardioversion.

     VFib: Cardioversion, lidocaine, procainamide, or bretylium.

     SVT: Adenosine, carotid sinus massage, Valsalva's maneuver, or verapamil.

     AFib: Digoxin or verapamil.

Pain

DEFINITION

Pain is defined as a noxious sensation. The term encompasses many types of discomfort, ache, and unpleasant perception, but not such sensations as nausea, dizziness, and pruritis. Doctors, often underestimate the value of pain control, but of all the advances in modern medicine, analgesia is one of the most reliable. You may be unable to cure a patient of cancer, but you can almost certainly relieve his pain.

TYPES OF PAIN

1. *Localized pain* occurs at the site of the injury or stimulus. A broken bone, for example, usually hurts at the exact site of the fracture.
2. *Referred pain* occurs at a site different from the injury or stimulus. Shoulder pain, for example, may be caused by a stimulus occurring under the diaphragm.
3. *Neuropathic pain* can be perceived at any site but is caused by damage or stimulus to the nerve rather than tissue damage of the perceived site.
4. *Phantom pain* is perceived as arising from a missing body part; it is caused by nerve stimulation.

MANAGEMENT

1. Focused history
   - Where does it hurt?
   - Severity
   - Quality: Sharp, dull, burning, aching, etc.
   - What instigates the pain? What relieves it?
   - Change with position, movement, inspiration, exertion, etc.
   - Time sequence: Abrupt, acute, chronic, intermit-

tent, constant, progressive, waxing and waning, episodic
- Trauma or other injury?

2. Focused physical examination
   - Tenderness? Sensitive to light touch, deep palpation?
   - Warmth, edema, redness?
   - Rebound phenomenon?
3. Focused diagnostic testing depends on site and differential diagnosis
4. Treatment
   - The best treatment is to remove the offending cause.
   - Nonpharmacologic treatment is often useful. Musculoskeletal injuries respond to cold during the first 24 hours and heat thereafter. Massage often works for muscle spasm. Rest is good for almost all types of pain.
   - The simplest analgesic is acetaminophen, which is safe, effective, and practically devoid of side effects when used in proper doses.
   - The next line of pharmacologic therapy is the nonsteroidal anti-inflammatory drugs. Examples include aspirin, ibuprofen, naproxen, and a host of others. Common side effects include gastrointestinal upset and renal damage.
   - The next line of treatment is the opioids. The simplest example is codeine, which is administered most conveniently in various combinations with acetaminophen. Intermediate-strength opioids include propoxyphene and oxycodone. High-strength opioids include morphine, hydromorphone, and levorphanol.

     Common side effects include sedation, nausea, and constipation.

     Habituation is a real problem but usually occurs after prolonged use, not after temporary treatment of acute pain.

- Local injection with anesthetics (such as lidocaine) and corticosteroids often provides long-lasting relief of chronic musculoskeletal pain.
- Nerve blocks are often used for chronic pain from cancer or other causes.
- Capsaicin, an agent derived from chili peppers, is applied as a topical creme and may be useful in treating musculoskeletal pain.

TIPS

For *chronic pain*, the tricyclic antidepressants may potentiate the action of other analgesics. Low doses often suffice.

For *persistent pain*, it is better to order analgesics as "around the clock—patient may refuse" rather than as "PRN." In the PRN order, the nurse will offer the medication only if the patient asks for it. In the "around the clock" order, the nurse will come to the patient and offer the medication. This avoids unnecessary delay and anxiety in analgesia.

A useful agent in chronic severe pain is the *fentanyl patch*, which releases a high-potency opioid through the skin over 72 hours. This has the advantage of providing steady blood levels rather than the peak and trough pattern of oral or injection dosing.

Continuous intravenous infusion is often used for severe pain, such as occurs after surgery or in cancer. The best example is a morphine infusion. A popular variant is known as *patient-controlled analgesia*, in which the patient controls the rate of the infusion from minute to minute.

The choice of *meperidine* as a high-potency opioid is popular but often ill-advised. The drug lowers the seizure threshold and interacts unfavorably with other agents, especially monoamine oxidase inhibitors.

For *acute abdominal pain*, analgesia is withheld until the precise diagnosis and therapy have been determined. Early analgesia may mask the acute process and prevent recognition of a life-threatening event.

Tempering this guideline with compassion may allow for some analgesia.

Pain that does not match a known pathophysiologic syndrome may reflect anxiety, depression, or somatization.

Ask your patients often about their pain. Pain control, when inadequate, can be improved by increasing the dose, frequency, or potency of the medication. Analgesia can be tapered later as the underlying condition improves.

Chest Pain

DEFINITION

Chest pain, simply enough, is pain in the chest. Many of the syndromes below can present as pain in the back or lateral chest.

DIFFERENTIAL DIAGNOSIS

1. Cardiovascular
   - Myocardium: MI, angina pectoris
   - Pericardium: Pericarditis
   - Great vessels: Aortic dissection
   - Valves: Mitral valve prolapse
2. Respiratory
   - Lung parenchyma: Pneumonia, neoplasm
   - Pleura: Pleuritis, pulmonary embolism, pneumothorax
   - Airway: Foreign body, aspiration
3. Gastrointestinal
   - Esophagus: Esophageal spasm, esophagitis, neoplasm
   - Stomach: Peptic ulcer, gastritis, neoplasm
   - Duodenum: Peptic ulcer, duodenitis
   - Gallbladder: Cholecystitis, biliary colic
4. Musculoskeletal
   - Ribs: Costochondritis, trauma
   - Intercostal muscles: Trauma, strain

5. Neurologic
   - Radiculopathy
   - Neuropathy

MANAGEMENT

1. Focused history
   - Quality of pain: Pressure, burning, sharp, dull?
   - Radiation, diaphoresis, nausea, lightheadedness
   - Precipitating and relieving factors. Exertional? Pleuritic? Positional? Relating to swallowing or eating? Prior occurrence?
   - Dyspnea? Cough?
   - Trauma?
2. Focused physical examination
   - Vital signs: BP, HR, and respiratory rate (RR)
   - Chest: Breath sounds, percussion
   - Cardiac: Jugular venous distention, gallop, rub, murmur, click?
   - Abdomen: Tenderness
   - Musculoskeletal: Are symptoms reproduced with palpation or with arm maneuvers?
   - Neurologic: Spine tenderness, zoster
3. Focused diagnostic testing
   - EKG
   - Chest x-ray
   - Consider response to therapeutic trial: Nitroglycerin, antacids
   - Consider: arterial blood gas
4. Treatment
   - If EKG demonstrates cardiac ischemia, treat for same. Classes of therapeutic agents include nitrates, beta blockers, calcium channel blockers, morphine, oxygen, and anticoagulants (aspirin, heparin, and thrombolytic agents). The sequence is as follows:
     - □ Oxygen.
     - □ Aspirin.
     - □ Nitroglycerin, given sublingually or topically

for stable angina; also given intravenously for infarction or unstable angina.

- Beta blockers or calcium channel blockers, as tolerated by BP and HR. The goal is to reduce the BP and HR to low normal levels.
- If these are inadequate to control symptoms, or if unstable angina is present, heparin is indicated.
- If infarction is present, thrombolytic therapy is indicated unless there is a specific contraindication. Age is not a contraindication.

- If a diagnosis is not apparent at the completion of the history, physical, EKG and chest x-ray, consider evaluation for gastrointestinal disease.

TIPS

Consider life-threatening conditions first: MI, pulmonary embolism, aortic dissection, pneumothorax

Chest pain that is reproducible on pressure is likely to be musculoskeletal in origin. However, an acute MI will sometimes cause chest wall tenderness.

"Cardiac enzymes" consist of creatine kinase (MB, MM and MB fractions), sometimes combined with LDH and SGOT. In conventional measurement, the results of this test are not available for 4 to 24 hours, limiting the test's utility in the acute setting. A new test of CK MB "subforms" may be available soon and promises earlier diagnosis of acute MI.

Dyspnea

DEFINITION

Dyspnea is defined as a sense of difficult or labored breathing. Blocked nasal passages and similar problems can interfere with breathing but are not considered to cause dyspnea if mouth breathing is normal.

DIFFERENTIAL DIAGNOSIS

1. Respiratory mechanics
   - Muscular: As in muscular dystrophy
   - Skeletal: As with multiple rib fractures
   - Neurologic: As with Guillain-Barré syndrome
   - Pneumothorax
   - Pleural effusion
   - Increased abdominal girth: As with ascites or severe obesity
2. Airways
   - Obstruction
   - Foreign body
   - Pharyngeal spasm or edema
   - Bronchospasm
3. Lung interstitium
   - Interstitial lung disease
   - Interstitial edema, as in congestive heart failure
   - Interstitial pneumonitis
   - Lymphangitic spread of neoplasm
4. Lung parenchyma
   - Pneumonia
   - Pulmonary edema
   - Alveolitis
   - Neoplasm
   - Emphysema
5. Pulmonary circulation
   - Pulmonary embolism
   - Pulmonary vasculitis
   - Pulmonary hypertension
6. Heart
   - Congestive heart failure
   - Mitral valve disease
   - Cardiac ischemia
   - Cardiac tamponade
   - Right-to-left shunt
7. Systemic
   - Anxiety
   - Exercise

- Anemia
- Decreased inhaled oxygen (e.g., at high altitude)

MANAGEMENT

1. Focused history
   - Onset: Abrupt, acute, subacute, chronic, progressive?
   - History of smoking?
   - Fever?
   - Prior occurrence?
   - Is chest pain present?
   - Precipitating and relieving factors. Exertional? Positional?
   - Cough? Productive?
   - Trauma?
2. Focused physical examination
   - Vital signs: BP, HR, and RR
   - Tracheal deviation?
   - Chest: Accessory muscles, breath sounds, percussion, chest wall tenderness, diaphragmatic excursion
   - Cardiac: Jugular venous distention, gallop, rub, murmur, click?
   - Extremities: Cyanosis?
3. Focused diagnostic testing
   - EKG
   - Chest x-ray
   - Consider: arterial blood gas
4. Treatment

   Evaluate for respiratory insufficiency. Altered mental status, extreme use of accessory muscles, gasping, extreme tachypnea, or severe cyanosis are signs of respiratory distress. Intubation and mechanical ventilation should be considered.

   - If mild to moderate respiratory findings are present, consider obtaining an arterial blood gas before treating.

- *Oxygen should be given for almost all conditions with dyspnea.* The exception is chronic obstructive pulmonary disease with chronic hypercarbia, in which oxygen can cause hypoventilation.
- Further treatment depends on the working diagnosis.

TIPS

Consider acute, life-threatening conditions first: MI, pulmonary embolus, pneumothorax, bronchospasm.

Subjective dyspnea without tachypnea generally indicates either central hypoventilation or a psychogenic cause.

Wheezing may be caused either by bronchospasm or pulmonary vascular congestion. When wheezing is present, look carefully for signs of congestive heart failure or of increased left ventricular end-diastolic pressure.

A frequently missed diagnosis is *pulmonary embolism*. When the cause of dyspnea is not apparent, consider this diagnosis seriously. Arterial blood gas is an important, if imperfect, test. An increased alveolar-arterial gradient, in the presence of a normal exam and chest x-ray, compels further workup.

Abdominal Pain

DEFINITION

Abdominal pain, simply enough, is pain localized to the abdomen.

DIFFERENTIAL DIAGNOSIS

Note that *neoplasm* and *trauma* can be added to each of the categories that follow.

1. Stomach
    - Gastritis
    - Ulcer
2. Proximal duodenum

    - Duodenitis
    - Ulcer
3. Gallbladder
    - Biliary colic
    - Acute cholecystitis
    - Cholangitis
4. Pancreas
    - Acute pancreatitis
    - Chronic pancreatitis
5. Bowels
    - Spasm
    - Inflammatory bowel disease
    - Enteritis (gastroenteritis)
    - Appendicitis
    - Ischemia
    - Strangulation
    - Bowel obstruction
    - Diverticulitis
    - Proctitis
6. Kidneys and ureters
    - Renal colic
    - Renal infarction
    - Pyelonephritis
7. Bladder
    - Infectious cystitis
    - Interstitial cystitis
8. Peritoneum
    - Perforated abdominal viscus
    - Peritonitis
9. Retroperitoneum
    - Aortic dissection
    - Hemorrhage
10. Miscellaneous
    - Endometriosis
    - Muscular pain
    - Referred pain from back
    - Referred pain from pelvis: Ovary, uterus, cervix, vagina, prostate

- Mesenteric adenitis: Can mimic appendicitis

MANAGEMENT

1. Focused history
   - All of the questions described under "Pain" previously are relevant.
   - Fever?
   - Relation to eating? to bowel movement? to urination?
   - Nausea or vomiting?
   - Blood in emesis, stool, or urine?
2. Focused physical examination
   - All of the findings described under "Pain" previously are relevant.
   - Observe patient position: supine? flexed at waist and hips? restive or still?
   - Bowel sounds: Increased, decreased, absent? high pitched?
   - Flank tenderness?
   - Pelvic examination should be considered.
   - *Murphy's sign*: Increased pain in the right upper quadrant with inspiration.
   - *Psoas sign*: Pain with leg elevation against resistance.
3. Focused diagnostic testing
   - CBC
   - Liver function tests and amylase
   - Abdominal x-ray
   - Urinalysis
   - Pregnancy test
   - Abdominal or pelvic sonogram
4. Treatment
   - Treatment depends entirely on the diagnostic impression.
   - Analgesia should not be given to a patient with acute abdominal pain until the evaluation has been completed and the diagnosis established.

This important principle must be tempered with compassionate regard for the patient's suffering.

TIPS

Consider acute, life-threatening conditions first: perforated viscus, peritonitis, strangulation, complete bowel obstruction, bowel ischemia, aortic dissection.

Pain that is initially relieved with food or antacid is likely to be *peptic* in nature, indicating some form of inflammation in the stomach or duodenum. The inflammation could reflect superficial irritation, ulcer, or neoplasm.

Gallbladder pain comes in three varieties. Biliary colic is intermittent and typically occurs after fatty meals. Acute cholecystitis begins abruptly, is more severe than colic, and does not necessarily follow meals. Cholangitis may be gradual in onset but is accompanied by fever and often a toxic appearance.

A patient with *pancreatitis*, whether acute or chronic, is restive and will often curl into a flexed position to relieve pressure in the retroperitoneum.

A *perforated viscus* is a medical emergency and is usually marked by absent bowel sounds, tachycardia, toxic appearance, and guarding. Glucocorticoids may mask these symptoms. An upright abdominal x-ray generally shows air under the diaphragm.

A hallmark of *peritonitis* is point tenderness with rebound. The patient avoids movement.

Appendicitis can mimic a great number of abdominal processes. One fairly consistent feature of appendicitis, however, is that it usually begins as pain (rather than nausea or fever).

Lower abdominal pain with rectal bleeding may be caused by ischemic colitis, ulcerative colitis, diverticulitis, enteritis, or proctitis. In patients who have taken broad-spectrum antibiotics, superinfection with *Clostridium difficile* can cause pseudomembranous colitis.

One of the great classics of diagnostic medicine is Zachary Cope's *The Early Diagnosis of the Acute Abdomen.*[1] First published in 1921, and still in print, neither time nor technology have lessened its value.

Acute Renal Failure

DEFINITION

Acute renal failure (ARF) is defined as an abrupt decline in kidney function. While there is no precise temporal cut-off, a decline in the creatinine clearance of 50% or more over several days or fewer should be considered ARF.

DIFFERENTIAL DIAGNOSIS

The causes of ARF can be categorized anatomically as prerenal, renal, or postrenal.

1. Prerenal
   - Systemic hypovolemia
   - Systemic hypotension
   - Renal artery stenosis (bilateral or unilateral with a solitary functioning kidney)
   - "Decreased effective renal perfusion" (edema states): Congestive heart failure, cirrhosis, hypoalbuminemia, and nephrotic syndrome
2. Renal
   - Glomerular: Glomerulonephritis, nephrotic syndrome
   - Interstitial/Tubular: Acute tubular necrosis (ATN), acute interstitial nephritis (AIN)
   - Vascular: Vasculitis, renal artery occlusion, renal vein thrombosis, cholesterol emboli syndrome, fat emboli syndrome
3. Postrenal

[1]Cope, Z: The Early Diagnosis of the Acute Abdomen, ed 6. London, Oxford University Press, 1932.

- Ureteral obstruction
- Bladder outlet obstruction
- Urethral obstruction

MANAGEMENT

1. Focused history
    - Oliguria
    - Hematuria
    - Drug
    - Chronic illness? (especially hypertension or diabetes)
    - Pain
2. Focused physical examination
    - Vital signs
    - Cardiovascular: Signs of congestive heart failure
    - Abdominal: Liver disease, ascites?
    - Flank tenderness
    - Bruit over aorta or renal artery
    - Suprapubic tenderness
    - Prostate
    - Edema
    - Skin: Eruption, vasculitis, collagen-vascular disease
    - Neurologic: Mental status, asterixis
3. Focused diagnostic testing
    - Electrolytes
    - BUN/Cr
    - Glucose
    - Urinalysis
    - Urinary sodium
    - Wright's stain of urine (To evaluate for eosinophils, the hallmark of AIN)
    - Abdominal sonogram
4. Treatment
    - Begin with localization of cause to prerenal, renal, or postrenal mechanism.

- In *prerenal* causes of ARF, increase fluids as tolerated

by clinical picture. Dopamine in a low-dose, continuous infusion is thought to increase renal blood flow in some patients.

- In *renal* causes of ARF, try to make the diagnosis by examining the urinary sediment.

  Granular casts imply ATN.
  RBC casts imply glomerulonephritis.
  Eosinophils on Wright's stain imply AIN.

  Then treat according to cause.
- In *postrenal* causes of ARF, relieve the obstruction. *Ureteral obstruction* is relieved by a nephrostomy tube or a ureteral stent. *Bladder outlet obstruction* or *urethral obstruction* is relieved by a suprapubic cystostomy or a Foley catheter.

TIPS

Localization is of the utmost importance and can be achieved with readily available clinical data.

The *hallmarks of prerenal azotemia* are:

- BUN/Cr ratio >20
- Elevated serum bicarbonate (contraction metabolic alkalosis)
- Oliguria
- Concentrated urine: Urine sodium ≤20 mEq/dL
- Hemoconcentration, as evidenced by a high hematocrit, uric acid, or albumin level

The *hallmarks of renal azotemia* are:

- Clinical setting consistent with glomerulonephritis or nephrotic syndrome
- Active sediment as described previously in "Treatment"
- On sonogram, the renal cortex is either swollen and heterogeneous (as in acute glomerulonephritis) or narrow and homogeneous (scarred, destroyed glomeruli).

The *hallmarks of postrenal azotemia* are:

- Hydronephrosis or hydroureter on sonogram
- Suprapubic tenderness or fullness, if distal obstruction is present
- High urine output after relief of the obstruction

The appearance of acute renal failure is often the new recognition of chronic renal failure, or slight deterioration of a chronic condition.

Renal damage in hospitalized patients is most often caused by:

- **Drugs.** Common offenders include aminoglycoside antibiotics, nonsteroidal anti-inflammatory agents, and radiographic contrast agents.
- *Inadequate renal perfusion*, due to excessive diuresis, inadequate fluid administration, or severe systemic illness.

Examining the urine yourself can be extremely useful. Routine laboratory urinalysis frequently misses such crucial findings as casts and abnormal cells.

A commonly overlooked cause of ARF is AIN, an allergic response that is frequently caused by penicillins and cephalosporins. The hallmark of AIN is the presence of eosinophils in the urine sediment; these can be found by performing a Wright's stain on the spun urine. The simplest way to obtain a Wright's stain is to prepare the unstained slide yourself, and then stain it with automatic equipment in the Hematology lab.

Altered Mental Status

DEFINITION

Altered mental status is defined as an impairment in mentation, arousal, consciousness, or awareness. Several different patterns should be distinguished.[2,3]

---

[2]Plum, F and Posner, JB: The Diagnosis of Stupor and Coma. Philadelphia, FA Davis, 1982.

[3]The Multi-Society Task Force on PVS: Medical aspects of the persistent vegetative state. N Engl J Med 1994;330:1499–1508.

- *Confusion* is a state of altered perception, understanding, or thought, with normal level of arousal.
- *Delirium* is a state of altered perception, understanding, or thought, with an increased level of arousal. Agitation, hyperexcitability, and hypervigilance are typically present; visual hallucinations may be present. Delirium is usually acute, temporary, and erratic.
- *Obtundation* is a state of reduced alertness, mild to moderate in degree, generally accompanied by drowsiness.
- *Stupor* is a deeper form of obtundation, with moderate to severe reduction in alertness, and frank sleepiness or sleep. The stuporous patient can be aroused but then lapses immediately into decreased responsiveness.
- *Coma* is a state of sustained unconsciousness, without awareness of self or environment, and without purposeful movement. Responses to stimuli may occur reflexively but not purposefully. The eyes remain closed, and there are no sleep-wake cycles. Breathing may be depressed but persists.
- *Persistent vegetative state* is a condition of sustained unconsciousness, without awareness of self or environment, but with sleep-wake cycles present.
- *Brain death* is an irreversible cessation of all brain functions. There is no spontaneous breathing, and no evidence of function at the brain stem or above. Spinal reflexes may be present.
- *Psychosis* is an inability to distinguish reality from unreality. It is characterized by delusions, hallucinations, and mental disorganization.
- *Dementia* is a progressive, organic decline in mental functioning. Multiple cognitive deficits, including memory impairment, are present.

DIFFERENTIAL DIAGNOSIS

Differential diagnosis for *acute* change in mental status begins by distinguishing causes intrinsic to the CNS from extrinsic processes.

1. Intrinsic
   - Vascular: Stroke, hemorrhage, hematoma, vasculitis
   - Trauma
   - Seizure
   - Tumor: Primary or metastatic
   - Infection: Meningitis, encephalitis
   - Cerebral edema, often associated with changes in serum osmolality
   - Psychosis
2. Extrinsic (also called "metabolic encephalopathy")
   - Hypoxia
   - Hypoglycemia
   - Cerebral hypoperfusion
   - Electrolyte disturbance: Sodium, potassium, calcium, magnesium
   - Renal failure
   - Hepatic insufficiency
   - Severe acidosis or alkalosis
   - Remote effect of fever or severe medical disease, especially infection
   - Thyroid dysfunction
   - Drug intoxication or other CNS effect
   - Drug or alcohol withdrawal
   - Vitamin deficiency, especially thiamin and B_{12}

MANAGEMENT

1. Focused history
   - Establish time course
   - Prior disturbance in mental status?
   - Psychiatric disease?
   - Trauma?
   - Medication or drug?
   - Loss of consciousness?
   - Abnormal or involuntary movements?
   - Acute or chronic medical illness?
2. Focused physical examination
   - Vital signs: Temperature, BP, HR
   - Neurologic examination: Focal or nonfocal

- Pupils
- Funduscopic examination: Papilledema?
- Signs of trauma: Skull ecchymosis, bony depression, blood or CSF in the ear canals or nares
- Nuchal rigidity?
- Asterixis?

3. Focused diagnostic testing
   - Electrolytes (including calcium and magnesium), creatinine
   - Glucose
   - Arterial blood gas
   - Consider: Serum ammonia, which is elevated in hepatic insufficiency; thyroid tests, vitamin B_{12} levels, and syphilis serology; and drug screen (blood or urine)
   - Head CT scan
4. Treatment
   - Identify whether the patient is breathing adequately and can protect the airway. If not, intubation is indicated.
   - If there are signs of increased intracranial pressure or uncal herniation, such as papilledema, Cushing's reflex, or pupillary asymmetry, treatment should consist of hyperventilation, mannitol, and possibly glucocorticoids.
   - If there is a focal abnormality on neurologic exam, a CT scan should be performed immediately.
   - If the diagnosis is not apparent from the history and physical exam, the patient should be given three agents as a matter of course:

     Glucose, to treat possible hypoglycemia

     Thiamine, to treat possible Wernicke's encephalopathy

     Naloxone, to treat possible opioid ingestion
   - If the diagnosis is still not apparent after simple blood tests have been performed, CT scan is indicated.

- Treatment of metabolic encephalopathy depends on the identification and correction of the underlying cause.

TIPS

Altered mental status is very common in hospitalized patients, especially the elderly and the very sick. The older the patient, the greater the chance of alteration in mental status during hospitalization. *Common causes in the elderly* include:

- Drug effect
- Remote effects of illness
- "Sundowning"—a phenomenon in which an older person becomes confused at night. Sundowning is attributed to a loss of the visual and auditory clues that occur during a bustling day.

Some acute metabolic encephalopathies, such as hypoxia, hypoglycemia, and cerebral hypoperfusion, cause irreparable CNS damage if not corrected promptly. These should always be considered first and treated immediately.

A common cause of altered mental status occurring on days 2 to 4 of hospitalization is *withdrawal* from alcohol or drugs, especially benzodiazepines.

Intrinsic CNS processes tend to lead to focal neurologic deficits; extrinsic processes lead to nonfocal deficits. However, an extrinsic process such as hypoglycemia can sometimes cause a focal deficit.

When mental status is impaired by metabolic processes, correcting the metabolic derangement may not correct mental status immediately. In general, the more insults to the CNS and the older the patient, the longer the recovery period from metabolic encephalopathy. An elderly patient with mild Alzheimer's disease who then develops renal insufficiency or hypercalcemia may not return to normal mental function until several days after these conditions have been corrected.

Persons who become confused or delirious often benefit from frequent orientation, reassurance, and calming.

What appears as an acute change in mental status may, in fact, reflect a chronic process that has worsened slightly, or that has become more noticeable to an occasional visitor. This is especially true of dementia. In evaluating an elderly patient with altered mental status, the patient's acquaintances should describe exactly what the patient could and could not do in the recent past: balance a checkbook, shop, prepare food, dress, toilet, etc.

Asterixis can be found in any metabolic encephalopathy but is most common in renal or hepatic insufficiency.

An important but often overlooked cause of obtundation or stupor is *status epilepticus*. If the diagnosis is unclear, a trial of intravenous diazepam may be warranted; improvement implies seizure.

Anemia

DEFINITION

Anemia is defined as a low level of hemoglobin. The normal range of hemoglobin is 14 to 18 g/dL in adult men, and 12 to 16 g/dL in adult women. Normal ranges in children are somewhat lower, depending on age.

The hematocrit is currently a calculated, hence derivative, value. Ordinarily, the hematocrit is about three times the hemoglobin, so that the normal range of the hematocrit is 42% to 54% in men and 36% to 48% in women.

DIFFERENTIAL DIAGNOSIS

1. Increased loss of RBCs
   - Bleeding
     - External hemorrhage

- Internal hemorrhage
- Surgical blood loss

- Hemolysis
  - Extrinsic to RBC
    - Artificial heart valves
    - Disseminated intravascular coagulation
    - Thrombotic thrombocytopenic purpura
    - Hemolytic uremic syndrome
    - RBC antibodies
  - Intrinsic to RBC
    - Abnormal RBC membrane: Hereditary spherocytosis, paroxysmal nocturnal hemoglobinuria
    - Abnormal hemoglobin: Thalassemia, sickle cell
    - Abnormal enzymes: G6PD (glucose-6-phosphate dehydrogenase) deficiency

2. Decreased production of RBC
   - Inadequate substrate
     - Iron deficiency
     - B_{12} deficiency
     - Folate deficiency
     - Thiamine deficiency
   - Bone marrow suppression
     - Uremia
     - "Chronic disease"
     - Hypothyroidism
     - Toxins: Alcohol, drugs
   - Bone marrow infiltration
     - Hematologic neoplasm
     - Metastatic malignancy
     - Amyloidosis
     - Granulomatous disease

MANAGEMENT

1. Focused history
   - Bleeding?
   - Recent surgery? Melena?

- Underlying medical conditions?
- Family history
- Medications or drugs? Alcohol?

2. Focused physical examination
   - Vital signs, including orthostatic blood pressure
   - Pallor
   - Lymphadenopathy
   - Splenomegaly
   - Stool guaiac
3. Focused diagnostic testing
   - CBC
   - Reticulocyte count
   - Examine peripheral blood smear
   - To assess iron status: Ferritin
   - B_{12} and folate
   - Serum creatinine
   - Consider: thyroid tests, bone marrow biopsy
   - If considering hemolysis: Coombs' test, haptoglobin
4. Treatment
   - *Transfusion* is indicated for:
     - Anemia plus symptoms, including chest pain, altered mental status, or extreme lassitude
     - Hgb <8 g/dL with no expectation of spontaneous improvement
     - Hgb <8 g/dL with coronary artery disease or with multiple risk factors
     - Rapidly falling hemoglobin with clinical evidence for hemorrhage
   - *Iron* is indicated only when iron deficiency has been documented, or when clear blood loss from a known cause has occurred.
   - When anemia is secondary to a nonhematologic disorder, the best treatment of the anemia is the treatment of the primary disorder.
   - Erythropoietin is useful in anemia due to renal insufficiency, and may be helpful in anemia due to AIDS or other chronic disease.

DIFFERENTIAL DIAGNOSIS

1. Respiratory
   - Chronic hypoxia from any cause
   - Sleep apnea
2. Cardiovascular
   - Congestive heart failure
   - Congenital heart disease
3. Gastrointestinal
   - Liver disease
   - Inflammatory bowel disease
   - Nutritional deficiency
4. Renal
   - Chronic renal insufficiency
   - Fluid or electrolyte disturbance
5. Hematologic
   - Anemia
   - Chronic hemolysis
6. Infectious
   - Infectious mononucleosis
   - Any chronic infection, including hepatitis, endocarditis, osteomyelitis, abscess, and HIV
7. Endocrine
   - Hyperthyroidism or hypothyroidism
   - Diabetes mellitus
   - Adrenal insufficiency or excess
8. Neoplasm
9. Collagen-vascular disorders
10. Psychogenic
    - Depression
    - Anxiety
    - Stress reaction
11. Drugs or medications
12. Chronic disease: Nearly any
13. *Chronic fatigue syndrome* (CFS) is a condition characterized by abnormal fatigue for ≥6 months, accompanied by fevers, lymphadenopathy, or sore throats, without primary depression or other

TIPS

After detecting anemia, the first step should be the *reticulocyte count* (retic). The retic is elevated in increased RBC loss and is normal or decreased in decreased RBC production.

Examination of the *peripheral smear* is often diagnostic. Remember that a normal MCV, as measured by a Coulter counter, may mask a mixed population of large and small RBCs. This should be reflected in an increased red cell distribution width.

If the retic is elevated, a Coombs' test and haptoglobin should be performed. A decreased haptoglobin confirms hemolysis. A positive Coombs' test indicates antibodies to RBC. LDH, although often invoked, is not a terribly useful test in evaluating hemolysis.

If the retic is normal or decreased, a ferritin and B_{12}/folate should be performed. If these are normal, consider thyroid tests and a bone marrow biopsy.

Anemia of chronic disease is common but should be inferred only when the retic is not elevated, a clear chronic disease has been identified, and results from diagnostic tests are unrevealing.

Giving iron indiscriminately to anyone with anemia is a bad idea. Iron works in iron deficiency and not otherwise.

Outpatient Problems

Fatigue

DEFINITION

Fatigue is described as an inordinate sense of tiredness. Fatigue is normal following exertion, stress, illness, or sleeplessness but should be relieved by rest. Persistent fatigue that is not relieved by adequate rest is abnormal.

known diagnosis. While most persons with persistent fatigue do not have CFS, the syndrome does appear to be a "real" and debilitating disease.

MANAGEMENT

1. Focused history
   - Underlying medical conditions
   - Constitutional symptoms: Fever, weight loss
   - Dyspnea?
   - Signs of depression?
   - Overwork? Inadequate rest? Stress?
2. Focused physical examination
   - Vital signs
   - Lymphadenopathy
   - Cardiovascular exam
   - Hepatosplenomegaly
   - Edema
   - Signs of thyroid dysfunction
3. Focused diagnostic testing
   - CBC
   - Biochemistry profile
   - Urinalysis
   - Thyroid tests
   - Consider: Sedimentation rate
4. Treatment
   - Depends on diagnosis.
   - Psychologic support is essential.

TIPS

The most common causes of fatigue are the triad of depression, anxiety and stress, on the one hand, and overwork on the other. Questions aimed at these hypotheses should be part of every evaluation for fatigue.

Medications that commonly cause fatigue include beta blockers, centrally acting alpha blockers, antihistamines, sedatives, antidepressants, neuroleptics, antiepileptics, and opioid analgesics.

In a person who appears well and whose physical examination and basic laboratory data are normal, a search for an occult malignancy only rarely bears fruit.

There is no general "pick-me-up" for fatigue. Remedies such as vitamin supplements, B_{12} injections, and iron are ineffective.

Lifestyle modification, or what the ancients used to call "regimen," is often helpful. Regular exercise, balanced diet, avoidance of "junk food," reduction of caffeine and alcohol, and adequate rest are often curative.

Hypertension

DEFINITION

Hypertension is defined as an abnormal elevation of BP. By convention, BP is elevated when the systolic pressure is ≥140 mm Hg or when the diastolic pressure is ≥90 mm Hg.

DIFFERENTIAL DIAGNOSIS

1. "Essential hypertension" (In 95% of cases, no cause identified)
2. Renal artery stenosis
3. Renal parenchymal disease
4. Hyperthyroidism
5. Pheochromocytoma
6. Cortisol excess (Cushing's syndrome)
7. Aldosterone excess (Conn's syndrome)
8. As a consequence of pain, anxiety, or exercise
9. As a consequence of medications, drugs, or alcohol

MANAGEMENT

1. Focused history
   - **Duration.** A diagnosis of chronic hypertension should not be made unless the blood pressure is

elevated on three different measurements, separated by at least 2 weeks.
- Acute secondary manifestations: Headache, visual disturbance, hematuria, or edema
- Chronic secondary manifestations: History of cerebrovascular, cardiovascular, or renal disease
- Episodic flushing or tachycardia
- Medications, drugs, and alcohol
- Life stressors

2. Focused physical examination
   - BP, taken after ≥5 minutes rest, in both arms
   - HR
   - Cardiovascular exam: Especially apical impulse, heart sounds, S_4, and peripheral pulses
   - Bruit over the aorta or renal arteries
   - Edema
3. Focused diagnostic testing
   - Electrolytes, BUN/Cr
   - Urinalysis
   - Thyroid tests
   - Serum catecholamines
   - **Renin.** This is most accurate when compared to 24-hour sodium excretion.
   - **Captopril test.** An exaggerated increase in plasma renin levels after the administration of captopril 25 mg suggests renovascular hypertension.
4. Treatment
   - If signs of acute secondary manifestations are present, hospitalization and prompt treatment are indicated. Blood pressure can be reduced in 15 to 60 minutes with the oral administration of some beta blockers and calcium channel blockers. More rapid reduction can be obtained by administering the same agents intravenously, or by intravenous infusions of nitroprusside, phentolamine, or esmolol.
   - If no signs of acute secondary manifestations are present, treatment is not urgent.

- Nonpharmacologic interventions for BP reduction include:
  - Weight loss, in the overweight. Highly effective.
  - Exercise, especially aerobic exercise.
  - Alcohol reduction to no more than two portions daily.
  - Salt reduction affords modest improvement, at best.
  - Dietary supplementation with calcium, magnesium, or potassium may be helpful.
  - Stress reduction is usually not a major factor.
- First-line agents for treating chronic hypertension include diuretics, beta blockers, calcium channel blockers, and angiotensin converting enzyme (ACE) inhibitors.
- When a single agent is inadequate in its maximal dose, a second first-line agent is added—usually a thiazide diuretic in small doses.
- Subsequent choices include peripheral alpha blockers and central alpha blockers. These are usually not given as monotherapy, since they cause reflex tachycardia.
- Third-line and fourth-line agents include methyldopa, minoxidil, hydralazine, and guanethidine.

TIPS

Acute secondary complications occur as a result of the BP at that time. *Chronic secondary complications* occur as a result of sustained hypertension. Most of the time, therapy is concerned with preventing chronic complications.

Acute secondary complications may occur at modest pressures in persons with chronic low pressure, and during pregnancy (toxemia).

A diagnostic search for the cause of hypertension is suggested if:

- The pressure is severely elevated.

- The pressure has increased rapidly.
- Systemic symptoms are present.
- Multiple endocrine neoplasia is suspected.
- A renal bruit is heard.
- Therapeutic efforts are unsuccessful.

A dramatic response to ACE inhibitors, especially in small doses, suggests renovascular hypertension.

The *initial choice of agent* depends on the clinical scenario. In persons with diabetes or decreased left ventricular function, ACE inhibitors are the agents of choice. In persons with coronary artery disease or left ventricular hypertrophy, beta-blockers and calcium channel blockers are preferred. In African Americans, thiazide diuretics may be best.

The elderly are susceptible to a syndrome called "isolated systolic hypertension," in which systolic pressure is ≥160 mm while diastolic pressure is <90 mm. Treatment, which had formerly been withheld in this syndrome, has recently been shown to be beneficial. Begin with either a thiazide diuretic or a beta blocker. If this is unsuccessful, switch to the other agent, or use both.

Agents that cause vasodilatation or orthostatic hypotension should be avoided in the elderly, if possible.

Drugs that can ***cause*** *hypertension* include decongestants, bronchodilators, oral contraceptives, other estrogens, androgens, glucocorticoids, excessive amounts of thyroxin, CNS stimulants, cocaine, and monoamine oxidase inhibitors. Chronic alcohol use, usually three or more portions daily, can also increase BP.

Cough

DEFINITION

Cough is defined as a forceful, explosive, usually involuntary exhalation.

DIFFERENTIAL DIAGNOSIS

1. Nasopharynx
    - Infection
    - Allergic rhinitis
    - Wegener's granulomatosis
    - Neoplasm
    - Foreign body
2. Oropharynx
    - Pharyngitis
    - Postnasal drip
    - Pertussis
    - Neoplasm
    - Foreign body
3. Trachea and airways
    - Tracheobronchitis
    - Neoplasm: Carcinoma, lymphoma
    - Chemical, thermal, or smoke inhalation
    - Aspiration
    - Tracheoesophageal fistula
    - Gastroesophageal reflux
    - Bronchospasm
    - Foreign body
4. Alveoli
    - Pneumonia.
    - Tuberculosis, a form of pneumonia, warrants specific mention.
    - Abscess.
    - Pneumonitis.
    - Neoplasm.
    - Pulmonary edema.
5. Interstitium
    - Interstitial pneumonitis
    - Interstitial edema
6. Pleura
    - Pleurisy and pleuritis
    - Pleural effusion and empyema
7. Diaphragm
    - Subpulmonic effusion

- Subphrenic abscess
8. Mechanism unknown
   - Drug effect, especially ACE inhibitors
   - "Psychogenic cough"

MANAGEMENT

1. Focused history
   - Time course
   - Fever
   - Dry or productive
   - Sputum: Color, blood, foul-smelling
   - Changed by position?
2. Focused physical examination
   - Vital signs
   - Oropharyngeal exam
   - Chest exam
   - Cardiovascular exam
3. Focused diagnostic testing
   - Chest x-ray
   - Spirometry
   - Direct laryngoscopy
4. Treatment depends on diagnosis

TIPS

On careful questioning, the patient will often be able to distinguish whether the cough arises from the nasopharynx, throat, or chest.

An acute productive cough, with little or no fever, generally indicates *tracheobronchitis*. Moderate or high fever, dyspnea, or a toxic appearance suggests *pneumonia*.

Foul-smelling sputum may indicate *abscess*.

Persistent, nonproductive cough that arises from the throat often indicates postnasal drip, one of the most common causes of chronic cough in adults.

Persistent cough that is nonproductive or productive of clear sputum is typical of asthma. Interstitial lung diseases, such as sarcoidosis, can present the same way.

Cough that is worse in the recumbent position may represent either congestive heart failure or gastroesophageal reflux. The latter is often accompanied by heartburn or by a sour taste on waking.

Joint Pain

DEFINITION

Joint pain, simply enough, is pain in a joint. Pain is described as *arthritis* when accompanied by signs of inflammation, such as swelling, erythema, and warmth. Pain without inflammation is called *arthralgia*. Patterns of joint involvement include:

- *Monoarthritis* in which a single joint is involved
- *Polyarthritis* in which two or more joints are involved. The term "*oligoarthritis*" is often used when a small number of joints, typically two to six, is involved.

DIFFERENTIAL DIAGNOSIS

1. Acute monoarthritis
   - Septic arthritis, including gonococcus
   - Acute gout
   - Pseudogout (calcium pyrophosphate crystal deposition disease)
   - Trauma
   - Hemarthrosis, as in hemophilia
   - Osteonecrosis
2. Chronic monoarthritis
   - Osteoarthritis.
   - Trauma.
   - Indolent infection, such as tuberculosis and fungus.
   - Gout and pseudogout may become chronic.

3. Polyarthritis
   - Collagen-vascular diseases: Lupus, rheumatoid arthritis, sarcoidosis, and others
   - Vasculitis
   - Endocarditis
   - Infection: Lyme disease, gonococcus, syphilis
   - Poststreptococcal infection (rheumatic fever)
   - During or after viral infections, especially hepatitis B
   - Serum sickness

MANAGEMENT

1. Focused history
   - Time course
   - History of trauma
   - Drug exposure
   - Fever
   - *Are symptoms worse in the morning or the evening?*
   - Stiffness
   - Distribution
   - Symptoms related to the eyes, urethra, or bowels
   - Family history
2. Focused physical examination
   - Temperature
   - General appearance
   - Joint exam: Edema, warmth, erythema, tenderness, effusion, range of motion, synovial thickening
   - Skin
3. Focused diagnostic testing
   - Joint aspiration
   - Serologies
   - CBC, sedimentation rate
4. Treatment depends on diagnosis. Nonspecific treatments consist of heat, rest, and acetaminophen or a nonsteroidal anti-inflammatory drug. Injection with local anesthetics and corticosteroids is often helpful, if there is no evidence of infection.

TIPS

Symmetric polyarthritis is most characteristic of collagen-vascular disorders.

A pattern of *morning stiffness* that is relieved by heat and motion typifies collagen-vascular disorders.

Joint pain with skin eruption or eye inflammation suggests collagen-vascular disease. Recent diarrhea or dysuria suggests Reiter's syndrome.

In acute monoarthritis, joint aspiration is indicated. The one possible exception is acute podagra, if all signs point to classic gout.

Polyarthralgia without inflammation often occurs during systemic illnesses, or in the aftermath of nonspecific viral syndromes. In the former case, they resolve with the illness; in the latter case, they may last for weeks to months before gradually fading and disappearing.

The conditions that usually cause polyarthritis can sometimes cause acute monoarthritis.

Oligoarthritis is most commonly seen in patients with Lyme disease, secondary syphilis, and sarcoidosis.

Rash

DEFINITION

Rash is defined as a skin eruption. Several patterns must be distinguished.

- *Macule*: a flat area with altered color. The skin surface is normal.
- *Patch*: a flat area with altered color and surface.
- *Papule*: a small, raised area, usually ≤5 mm in diameter and depth.
- *Nodule*: a larger raised area, usually >5 mm in diameter and depth.
- *Plaque*: a raised superficial area, usually >5 mm in diameter but shallow.
- *Cyst*: a nodule filled with fluid.

- *Vesicle*: a small, raised fluid collection in the superficial layers of skin, either within or just beneath the epidermis, usually ≤5 mm in diameter.
- *Bulla*: the same as a vesicle but >5 mm in diameter.
- *Pustule*: a vesicle that is filled with purulent material.
- *Wheal*: a localized area of edema in the dermis.
- *Telangiectasia*: a lacy branching pattern or tangle of dilated capillaries.

DIFFERENTIAL DIAGNOSIS

The most important syndromes are underlined.

1. Macular eruptions
   - **Erythema.** Erythematous eruptions that are purely macular are uncommon; they are more typically maculopapular, and are described below.
   - Hypopigmentation
     - *Vitiligo:* Sharply demarcated areas of complete depigmentation that may become confluent
     - *Postinflammatory:* Areas of relative pigment loss in areas of prior inflammation or injury
2. Maculopapular eruptions
   - Viral infection
     - <u>**Measles.**</u> Numerous red macules and papules begin on the face and then proceed downward, involving the trunk and then the entire body. Lesions often become confluent, especially on the face. Pruritis is mild to moderate.
     - **Rubella.** The lesions are similar to measles but typically less red. Confluence is less common.
     - <u>**Chickenpox**</u> **(Varicella).** The eruption starts on the trunk and then spreads to the limbs and head. Lesions begin as macules that progress to papules and then vesicles. Pruritis is moderate to severe.
     - **Shingles.** A macular, papular, or vesicular eruption in a dermatomal pattern, usually on the trunk, thigh, or head.

- **Roseola infantum (Exanthem Subitum).** Young children develop high fever followed by a macular or maculopapular eruption on the neck and trunk, possibly extending to the thighs and buttocks.
- **Fifth Disease (Erythema Infectiosum).** In children, a maculopapular eruption occurs on the limbs and trunk, typically following a period of mild fever and bright-red cheeks.
- **Other Viruses.** Macular or maculopapular eruptions can occur during infection with enteroviruses, Epstein-Barr virus, cytomegalovirus, adenovirus, HIV, and a number of others.

- Other infections
  - **Mycoplasma.** A generalized maculopapular eruption, more common in children.
  - **Rocky Mountain Spotted Fever.** After 2 to 6 days of high fever, a macular eruption begins on the distal limbs and then moves centrally, becoming maculopapular and often confluent.
  - **Typhoid Fever.** Small rose-colored papules occur on the chest and abdomen.
  - Streptococcus and Staphylococcus infections may cause a maculopapular eruption due to the release of toxins.
- **Allergic Reaction.** A measles-like ("morbilliform") eruption occurs frequently as a hypersensitivity reaction to many drugs and foods. The typical location is the upper chest or back, although any area may be involved.
- **Systemic Lupus.** A maculopapular eruption, often with telangiectasia, occurs in the classic malar distribution or in sun-exposed areas.

3. Papular eruptions
   - **Vasculitis.** Papules, often confluent, are typically palpable purpura, deep violaceous raised areas that do not blanch.
   - **Insect Bite.** Papules occur singly or in groups, often with local erythema or edema.

- **Scabies.** Numerous, tiny and intensely pruritic papules occur at virtually any site. On close examination, a minuscule burrow may be visible, especially in the finger web.
- **Miliaria (Heat Rash).** Small inflammatory papules occur in areas of skin that are warm and moist, especially when occluded by diapers, dressings, or bed linens.
- **Lichen Planus.** Plateau-shaped, pruritic, violaceous papules occur, often in linear streaks, on the wrists or other areas.
- Some of the miscellaneous infections that typically cause maculopapular eruptions can cause purely papular eruptions.

4. **Nodules.** Nodules are not eruptions in the strict sense but warrant attention. Common causes include neoplasm, wart, neurofibroma, and dermatofibroma.
5. Vesicles
   - **Herpes Simplex.** Grouped, painful vesicles occur on a red base.
   - **Herpes Zoster.** See "Shingles."
   - **Dermatitis Hepatiformis.** Groups of vesicles or bullae, severely pruritic, occur on the elbows, knees, or back.
   - **Contact Dermatitis.** Vesicles or bullae, often surrounded by erythema and edema, occur after direct contact with noxious substances. The prototype is poison ivy.
6. Bullae (see also "Vesicles")
   - **Pemphigus Vulgaris.** Superficial bullae occur on the buccal mucosa or elsewhere. They are not tense and break readily. Large areas of skin can become denuded, often becoming superinfected.
   - **Bullous Pemphigoid.** Large, tense bullae occur in the axilla, inguinal area, and areas of skin flexion.
   - **Porphyria Cutanea Tarda.** Bullae occur on the

back of the hands as a result of inborn errors in heme synthesis, often precipitated by alcohol or medications.
- **Bullous Impetigo.** Bullae form as a consequence of *Staphylococcus aureus* infection.
- **Toxic Epidermal Necrolysis.** Large bullae form and slough, usually due to a drug reaction.
- Common blisters are localized to areas of friction, especially the hands and feet.

7. Patches
   - **Cellulitis.** Bacterial infection in the skin causes circumscribed areas of erythema, warmth, edema, and tenderness, with no epidermal changes or with slight scaling.
   - **Tinea Versicolor.** Small areas of decreased pigmentation with fine scaling and variable color occur as a result of skin infection with a fungus, Pityrosporum.
   - **Pityriasis Alba.** Irregular patches of decreased pigmentation occur on the face or upper arm.
8. Plaques
   - **Eczema.** Raised areas of erythema, often accompanied by papules or vesicles. Common forms include:
     - **Atopic Dermatitis.** Pruritic plaques occur in persons with other allergies, as allergic rhinitis or asthma, on the hands, arms, neck, or elsewhere.
     - **Lichen Simplex Chronicus.** Sharply demarcated plaques occur as a result of persistent scratching.
     - **Seborrheic Dermatitis.** Scaling erythematous plaques, not sharply demarcated, occur in or near the scalp, or between the eyebrows, as an inflammatory reaction to oils.
     - **Idiopathic.** Pruritic plaques occur, nearly anywhere, without identifiable cause.
   - **Psoriasis.** Raised areas with erythema and

prominent white or silver scaling, often sharply circumscribed, occur on the elbows, knees, scalp, intragluteal cleft, or other areas.

- **Tinea.** Superficial fungal infections occur on the body (tinea corporis, ringworm), groin (tinea cruris), feet (tinea pedis), scalp (tinea capitis), or other areas. The lesions are raised, erythematous, scaly, sometimes annular, and pruritic.
- **Pityriasis Rosea.** A single, large, pink, oval plaque on the neck, trunk, or proximal limbs, the "herald patch," is followed by numerous smaller plaques that follow the skin lines.
- **Secondary Syphilis.** Small violaceous plaques or papules predominate on the palms and soles but may affect any area.
- **Discoid Lupus.** Red, ovoid, scaling plaques occur on the face and other sun-exposed areas.
- **Mycosis Fungoides.** These irregular red plaques or patches often occur on the back and are a cutaneous T-cell lymphoma.

9. Pustules
   - **Acne.** Inflammatory pustules, often with white or blackened domes, occur in areas of sebaceous glands.
   - **Rosacea.** Pustules and papules occur on an erythematous base, especially on the central face and nasolabial folds. Telangiectasias are typical.
   - **Folliculitis.** These small pustules have a hair in their centers and arise from mildly infected hair follicles.
   - **Impetigo.** Pustules, caused by Staph or Strep infection, break to form a characteristic honey-golden crust.
   - **Disseminated Infection (Bacteria, Fungus).** Embolized bacteria appear as numerous discrete pustules, especially on the limbs.
10. Other eruptions
   - **Erythema Multiforme.** Variable and consists of

erythematous macules, plaques, or bullae. The characteristic finding is the target lesion, a bull's-eye pattern of a central area that is red, dark, or vesicular, surrounded by a pale ring, which is surrounded by a raised red rim.
- **Urticaria.** Consists of one or more wheals that often have large plaques with pale centers.

MANAGEMENT

1. Focused history
   - Fever?
   - Other acute or chronic illness
   - Medications or other ingestions
   - Topical exposures
   - Pruritis
2. Focused physical examination
   - Temperature
   - General appearance
   - Description of lesion: Size, shape, color, surface appearance, and location
   - Distribution
3. Focused diagnostic testing
   - Scaling lesions should be scraped and examined under potassium hydroxide; hyphae indicate fungal infection.
   - Biopsy is often indicated.
   - Serologic tests or cultures are helpful in infectious diseases.
4. Treatment depends on diagnosis. While topical corticosteroids are effective in many dermatologic disorders, serious diagnoses can be missed if insufficient attention is given to accurate diagnosis.

TIPS

Describing skin lesions accurately is the biggest single step in diagnosis.

If a lesion blanches, blood remains in the capillaries. Absence of blanching indicates leaching of blood outside the capillaries.

Common causes of rash in hospitalized patients include drug reaction, cellulitis, and milia. In immunocompromised patients, disseminated infections such as cytomegalovirus, varicella, staphylococcus, Gram-negative bacilli, mycobacteria, fungus, and others should be considered.

PART III

THE DIAGNOSTIC PROCESS

CHAPTER 14

The Problem List

Clinical Problem Solving

1. Clinical diagnosis begins, of course, with the History and Physical Examination. Medical school courses often imply, incorrectly, that one should first perform a complete history, then perform a complete physical examination, and then begin to think about diagnosis. In fact, one begins to think about diagnosis from the very start. The skilled clinician forms diagnostic hypotheses early, often as early as the chief complaint. These hypotheses become the basis for further questions and examination maneuvers. As the interview and examination proceed, the clinician develops hypotheses, tests them via question and maneuver, and then decides whether to accept, to reject, or to revise them.
2. This means that the history and physical are often intermingled. The expert clinician does not ask every question and perform every examination technique for every patient. Rather, these are selected according to the physician's ability to test the developing hypotheses. If a history of increased urination is elicited, consider possible causes: cystitis, diabetes mellitus, diabetes insipidus, or prostatic hypertrophy. Then ask questions addressed to each

of these possibilities: dysuria, polydipsia and polyphagia, copious pale urine, or hesitancy and straining. Similarly, a physical finding of moist pulmonary crackles should lead to an assiduous search for congestive heart failure: jugular venous distention, cardiomegaly, hepatojugular reflux, and dependent edema. Choose questions and maneuvers, as much as possible, according to an idea. Examining for Chvostek's sign (facial contraction caused by tapping of the facial nerve) is important only when hypocalcemia or hypomagnesemia is being considered, and not otherwise.

3. Diagnostic thinking is often a reiterative process:
   - Elicit data (by history, physical, or laboratory)
   - Form a hypothesis
   - Gather new data (by history, physical, or laboratory) that tend to confirm or refute the hypothesis
   - Accept, reject, or revise the hypothesis
   - Consider: Has threshold for action been reached?
     If yes → act.
     If no → repeat these steps until the threshold has been reached.

4. The question often arises, "How complete should the history and physical be?" The degree of completeness varies according to the following:
   - The clinical problems at hand: What are the major issues?
   - The clinical setting: Hospital floor, outpatient practice, Emergency Department, Intensive Care Unit.
   - Urgency: Conditions that threaten life or limb imminently outweigh all else.
   - The patient's agenda: What the patient wants or expects of the encounter. A woman with a newly broken ankle may not benefit from a first-visit discussion of smoking cessation. However, she

may benefit when she returns for an annual health evaluation 2 months later.

5. Clinical problem solving is methodical. Experienced clinicians do not diagnose by intuition, nor by magic. Rather, they proceed stepwise through an algorithm that is simple in concept, although often complex in execution.
   - Problem list
   - Differential diagnosis
   - Diagnostic testing
   - Diagnosis
   - Therapy

The Problem List: General Principles

1. The *problem list* is an organized enumeration of relevant clinical data. It translates the hodgepodge of patient findings into discrete, recognizable quanta. The problem list has three functions:
   - To keep a roster of clinical data—such as you might keep on a notepad
   - To codify data—organizing data into major and subsidiary points (files and subfiles)
   - To track clinical data—marking the issues for subsequent reference
2. A *problem* is any clinical issue, a data point. There are seven main types of problems:
   - **A Symptom.** A *symptom* is anything that the patient observes, feels, or senses. In Alvan Feinstein's succinct definition, a symptom is "a subjective sensation or other observation that a patient reports about his body or its products."[1]

---

[1]Feinstein AR: Clinical Judgment. Baltimore, Williams & Wilkins, 1967.

- **A Sign.** A *sign* is anything that the examiner observes, "an entity objectively observed by the clinician during physical examination of the patient."
- **A laboratory value** or **test result**
- **A Prevalence-Modifier.** This is any feature of the patient that affects the prevalence of illnesses.
  - Habits: Tobacco, alcohol, drugs

    > ***Example:*** Smoking is a problem, because it increases the risk of several diseases.

  - Behavior that affects the risk of disease: Dietary, sexual, occupational, recreational, travel.

    > ***Example:*** Recent travel to Nantucket may be a problem, because it increases the risk of babesiosis.

  - Exposure to a disease or a disease vector

    > ***Example:*** Living with a person with TB is a problem, because it increases the risk of contracting TB.

  - Demographic feature

    > ***Example:*** Being a Pima Indian may be a problem, because the risk of diabetes is increased.

  - Family history

    > ***Example:*** A family history of colon cancer may be a problem, because it increases the risk of this disease.

  - Other susceptibility or proclivity

    > ***Example:*** Living in an area where an outbreak has occurred may be a problem, be-

cause it increases the possibility of exposure to a particular disease.

- **A Patient Opinion or Belief.** Might affect a patient's care.

  Examples

  A patient's conviction regarding diagnoses ("I must have cancer.")

  A patient's conviction regarding therapy ("Whenever I take aspirin, my toenails itch.")

  Treatments that are unacceptable to the patient (blood transfusions in Jehovah's Witnesses, pork insulin in some orthodox Jews)

  Personal, social, or ethnic models of disease

- **A Characteristic Cluster of Findings.** If a set of clinical findings form a compelling pattern, this may itself be identified as a problem.

  Example: In a patient with fever, new murmur, and splinter hemorrhages, "possible endocarditis" becomes a problem.

- **Prior Diagnosis or Known Medical Condition.** These should also be listed.

  Examples: Hypertension, history of splenectomy, history of nephrotic syndrome

3. A problem need not have a negative connotation. However, it does indicate that something is abnormal, or noteworthy, or out of the ordinary.
4. The challenge is to give shape to an unwieldy body of information. The history, physical examination, and laboratory data provide a (potentially) complete enumeration of patient data. These data are initially unformed and theoretically infinite. The problem list seeks to structure clinical data in a manageable form.

5. Problems may have different types of significance, according to whether they cause symptoms, or threaten health, or both.

   - Produces symptoms but does not signify serious illness

     Examples: Viral gastroenteritis, costochondritis

   - Signifies a possible serious illness but does not produce symptoms

     Examples: Mole, prostate nodule

   - Produces symptoms, and may signify serious illness

     Examples: Crushing chest pain, aphasia

   - Produces symptoms that the patient, but not the clinician, regards as problematic

     Example: Male balding

   Note that the boundary between "medical" and "nonmedical," like the northern limit of the Roman Empire, tends to shift.

Making the Problem List

1. **Generate.** Write down the salient features of the case (notepad function). Go through the history, examination, and laboratory data and write down anything that seems noteworthy.
2. **Translate.** Recast the patient's words, to the extent that accuracy allows, into medical terms. If the chief complaint was "I had a blackout," you should

know by the end of the history whether this meant loss of consciousness (coded as "syncope"), or feeling faint ("lightheadedness"), or a sense of abnormal movement ("vertigo.")

It is important to be as accurate as the patient data allow, neither more nor less. If the patient cannot really recall precisely whether the arm was weak or numb, the item should be coded as "arm symptoms."

3. **Lump and Split.** Lumping and splitting refers to the grouping of items on the problem list. Items that seem to go together are "lumped" as a single problem. Items that seem not to go together are "split" into separate problems.

Example

A patient has an early, high-pitched diastolic murmur, S_3 gallop, water-hammer pulse, head-bobbing, booming pulsations over the femoral arteries, and fingernail capillary pulsations. These findings can be lumped together as "probable aortic regurgitation."

Example

A patient with known cholelithiasis and occasional biliary colic develops severe pain in the left lower quadrant accompanied by fever and diarrhea. These findings should be split and entered separately as "cholelithiasis" and "left lower quadrant pain."

Lumping and splitting is not always obvious. What is at stake is the organization of clinical data along pathophysiologic principles. This process therefore involves making hypotheses about what is happening physiologically. These hypotheses should be considered provisional, not definitive. If a given organization of the problem list is not proceeding to a diagnosis, consider reorganizing the list.

Example

> A 28-year-old man, previously well, developed nausea and fatigue for 3 mos. Physical examination detected jaundice and splenomegaly. The peripheral blood smear demonstrated microspherocytes, leading to a diagnosis of hereditary spherocytosis. However, only after symptoms persisted for several months was a sample of stool examined; this demonstrated *G lamblia.* The failure to consider Giardia previously arose from the lumping of "nausea" together with the other clinical features. While this lumping made sense provisionally, it should have been reevaluated promptly as the patient's symptoms persisted.

4. **Rank.** Problems should be sorted according to their importance. Problems receive greater priority, and appear higher on the list, to the extent that they:
   - Threaten life and limb

     > ***Example:*** Acute dyspnea would appear high on the problem list

   - Require timely action

     > ***Example:*** Acute dyspnea would appear higher on the list than a breast mass. Although both are potentially life-threatening, the dyspnea requires immediate action.

   - Provide critical or discriminating information

     > ***Example:*** Mild back pain is a common and nonspecific finding that often merits low priority. When accompanied by focal motor weakness, however, it moves up on the problem list and receives increased priority.

- Are considered important by the patient

> ***Example:*** A patient who reports bitemporal headaches once weekly for 6 yr is also found to have mild mitral regurgitation, an enlarged ovary, and anemia. If the headaches are her first concern, they should go higher on the problem list than if they are only mentioned in passing.

5. **Edit.** Go back through the list, rechecking that you have included all pertinent data and that the organization makes sense.
6. When the problem list is complete, you have framed the clinical issues and defined the field of inquiry. You are ready for the next step, differential diagnosis.

CHAPTER 15

Differential Diagnosis

General Principles

Differential diagnosis involves the identification of the possible diagnoses for a given symptom, sign, clinical finding, or illness. The term is used to refer to three related concepts: to the list of possible diagnoses, to the list of alternative diagnoses, and to the *process* of finding possible diagnoses. In the first usage, one might say that the differential diagnosis of abdominal pain includes peptic ulcer, biliary colic, pancreatitis, etc. In the second, one might say that the differential diagnosis of acute cholecystitis includes acute pancreatitis ("the list of what it ain't"). In the third, one might say that the differential diagnosis of abdominal pain begins with localization, etc.

> Differential diagnosis is a way of generating hypotheses regarding the identity and cause of an illness. It is not an end in itself, but rather a route to the target, diagnosis.

For any given clinical finding, it is easy to think of a cause or two. Differential diagnosis involves a more comprehensive consideration of potential causes. This search for comprehensiveness requires a method for navigating the sea of clinical possibilities. The ideal method would be:

- Complete—every diagnosis can be reached through the method
- Conceptually simple (even if detailed)
- Structured—so that related entries can be considered and filed as a chunk

Strategies for Differential Diagnosis

There are seven principal methods for differential diagnosis. They vary in the degree to which they approximate the ideals described previously, and in their applicability for various contexts. While no one method is effective for all clinical problems, each is useful in the appropriate place.

Method 1. "What Crosses My Mind"

This is the most frequently used method for differential diagnosis, and the shoddiest. The vague clinician identifies a problem, names a few causes, performs perhaps a few tests, and then prescribes a treatment. "The patient has anemia, she must have iron deficiency, give her iron"—so goes the unarticulated deduction. It is worth mentioning because it is so widely encountered, and because it signals a kind of mental exhaustion or surrender. Be on guard, in yourself and in others.

Method 2. The Brilliant Guess

The brilliant guess is most popular on Morning Rounds, when a patient with enlarged lymph nodes is presented, and an enterprising intern blurts out, "Angioimmunoblastic lymphadenopathy!" Now, the patient could, in fact, have angioimmunoblastic lymphadenopathy; if so, the intern will look like a genius. But most of the time the patient will have something else, and the intern is left with nothing. The trouble with the brilliant guess is that it fails, even when correct, to provide a route from the problem list to the diagnosis; it leaps, as if magically. Serendipity is *not* a reliable strategy.

Method 3. The Simple List

A simple list is often the most succinct way to get from here to there. For example, the substances that, when ingested, can cause an anion-gap metabolic acidosis are aspirin, methanol, ethylene glycol, and paraldehyde. There it is. There is no way to retrieve this list other than to remember it or to write it down somewhere. Simple lists are most useful when they are short and when no other system of categorization exists. One renowned text of differential diagnosis provides a list of some 300 causes of abdominal pain—complete, to be sure, but not terribly helpful.

Method 4. The Mnemonic Device

Mnemonic devices are techniques for remembering. They usually take the first letter of each item on a list and make a catchy term or phrase. "On old Olympus' towering tops . . ."—thus the freshman medical student memorizes the cranial nerves, ophthalmic, otic, oculomotor, trochanteric, trigeminal, etc. The group of microorganisms that cause infectious endocarditis with negative blood cultures are often known as the HACEK organisms: *Hemophilus parainfluenzae, Actinobacillus actinomycetemcomitans, Cardiobacterium hominis, Eikenella corrodens,* and *Kingella* species. These little contraptions are useful—when used sparingly. In the case of the HACEK organisms, I know of no other way to remember the group. But there is, of course, no guarantee that you will not substitute *Acinetobacter* for *Actinobacillus*, or *Klebsiella* for *Kingella*. The problem is that mnemonic devices are based on an *arbitrary* system of classification, one without reference to pathophysiology. This resembles those libraries in which all the books with red covers sit on one shelf; items are classified according to their accidental properties rather than essential properties. One of the hallmarks of modern medicine is that disease has been organized according to pathophysiologic principles. These same principles should guide differential diagnosis.

Method 5. The Diagnostic Template

The diagnostic template is the first method we have considered that depends on *medical* thinking, as opposed to some other type of process. A template is a pattern that can be used repetitively as circumstances demand. A diagnostic template is essentially an outline of a clinical condition, structured according to medical concepts.

Renal failure, for example, can be due to renal, prerenal, or postrenal causes.

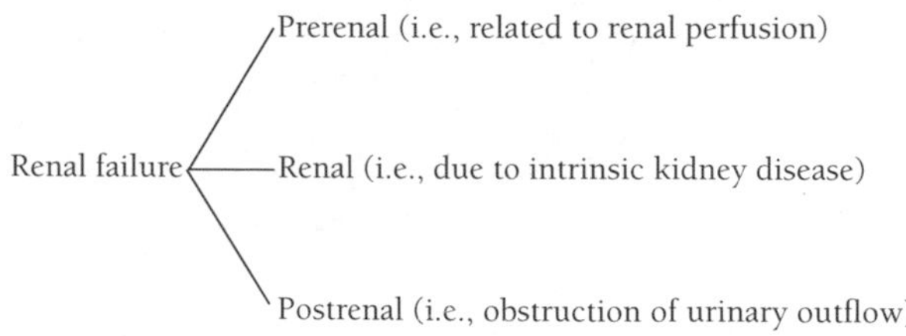

The division into three categories is based on an anatomic principle, namely that the cause of renal failure can be localized to three anatomic domains. Continuing, each of the three domains can be further divided into subsets.

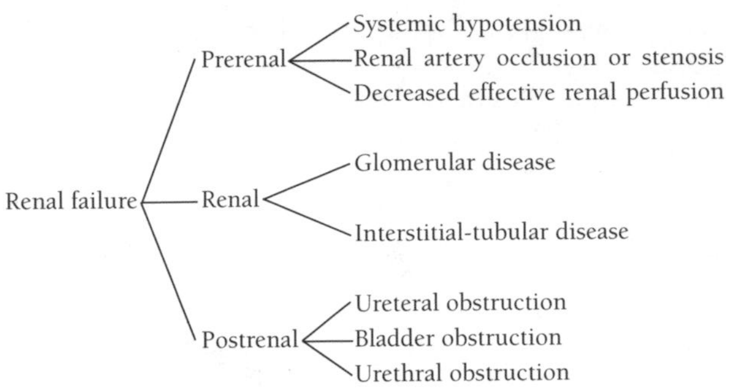

At each division, an anatomic principle creates a mental outline of the disease. This is fundamentally different from listing all the renal diseases that begin with the letter "C."

There are three advantages to thinking about diagnosis using templates:

1. Diagnostic reasoning is organized along medical principles. You are thinking medically, rather than straining memory banks.
2. The diagnostic template can be reconstructed on demand. If you make a template for a clinical problem once, you can recall and recreate it any time the problem arises.
3. The template can be constructed so that each branch point corresponds to a readily ascertainable fact.

Example

In renal failure, the question of prerenal azotemia can be decided by the BP, the BUN/Cr ratio, the serum bicarbonate level, and the urinary sodium level. The question of postrenal azotemia can be decided by a sonogram. If these are normal, the cause is renal azotemia. This point is inestimably valuable in performing differential diagnosis. If the sonogram is normal, you don't need to think any further (provisionally) about the ureters, bladder, prostate, or urethra. The field of possible diagnoses can be quickly narrowed.

Diagnostic templates can take advantage of two different ways of organizing the body: anatomy and pathophysiology. *Anatomic* classification can use several different levels of anatomic detail.

Gross anatomy

Example: Dysphagia: oropharynx, pharynx, esophagus, stomach

Tissue

Example: Proteinuria: glomerular, tubular

Cell

Example: Non-Hodgkin's lymphoma: B-cell or T-cell

Molecular

Example: Hemolysis: abnormal hemoglobin, normal hemoglobin

The second major design uses *pathophysiology* to structure the template.

Anemia: Due to increased erythrocyte destruction/loss or decreased erythrocyte production

Urticaria: Immunoglobulin-E–mediated, complement-mediated, nonimmunologic, idiopathic

Coagulopathy: Dysfunction of platelets, coagulation proteins, or vascular endothelium

Peripheral Edema: Volume overload, venous/lymphatic obstruction, capillary leak, decreased colloid osmotic pressure

Again, simple clinical facts can guide the diagnostic process by supporting, or excluding, diagnostic categories. In the differential diagnosis of anemia, the presence of increased reticulocytes excludes the category *decreased erythrocyte production* and indicates *increased erythrocyte destruction or loss.* This means that none of the causes of decreased erythrocyte production, including iron deficiency, B_{12} malabsorption, hypothyroidism, etc., need to be considered. In the differential diagnosis of abnormal bleeding, a normal bleeding time excludes *platelet dysfunction* as a possible cause.

The templates can be portrayed in two ways. The format given previously is a kind of decision tree, in which each division corresponds to an anatomic or pathophysiologic distinction. Alternately, the template can be portrayed as an outline, with each division corresponding to a subheading. The tree version helps to diagram your thought process; the outline version is more compact. Both work.

The diagnostic template is reusable. Sometime in your third year you will encounter a patient with jaundice. Make a diagnostic template for jaundice, and write it down somewhere; a pocket notebook is ideal. Then, the next time you meet a jaundiced patient, you can refer to your initial template. The data have changed, but the template remains the same. You need only plug in the new data.

Diagnostic templates provide a strategy for solving complex diagnostic puzzles. A 5-year-old boy has new renal failure and hemolytic anemia. First, make a diagnostic template for each problem. Then, look for points of intersection. If the previous outlines are completed, the points of intersection are found to be autoimmune disease (e.g., systemic lupus), vasculitis, and hemolytic-uremic syndrome. Diagnostic testing can focus on these entities.

Method 6. Cluster Recognition

Diseases and syndromes are distinctive patterns of clinical findings. If you can recognize a compelling pattern in a patient's symptoms, signs, or laboratory data, you have reached the (possible) diagnosis. Cluster recognition consists of choosing the chief points in a clinical scenario, connecting them, and associating them with a known disease or syndrome.

Cluster recognition borrows from Gestalt theory, a psychologic discipline that states that a shape is often perceived as an integrated whole rather than as the sum of its parts. A gosling identifies the shadow of a hawk at a glance, without scrutinizing whether the angle of the wing is more consistent with a pigeon. If you are deciding whether the person approaching you on the sidewalk may be your sister, you don't ruminate whether the nose is the right size, or the hair the right degree of curliness: you see in a flash that the person is Peggy, or not.

A young woman with nausea, fatigue, and secondary amenorrhea is likely to be pregnant. These findings form a clinical pattern that is most consistent with pregnancy. Now, it would certainly be possible to make a diagnostic template for secondary amenorrhea, and another for nausea, and then to find their points of intersection. Pregnancy would be one such point. However, if you can see the pattern of pregnancy, you can save yourself much labor and proceed directly to a likely hypothesis. Similarly, a man with high fever, headache, myalgia, and a macular eruption on the distal extremities is likely to have Rocky Mountain spotted fever (RMSF). These data points form the constellation of RMSF. The constellation of fever, renal insufficiency, hemolysis, thrombocytopenia, and neurologic changes constitutes thrombotic thrombocytopenic purpura until proven otherwise.

One difficulty in cluster recognition lies in the way the data points are chosen. A young man has bloody diarrhea after travel to Guatemala; these three points form the pattern of bacterial dysentery.

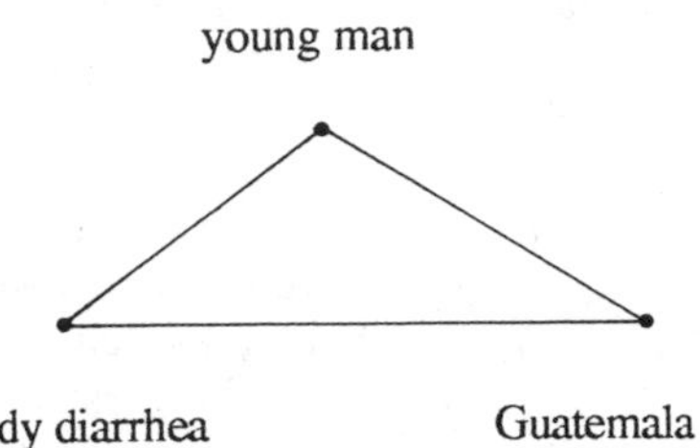

A second young man has bloody diarrhea in recurrent episodes over 4 years; these three points form the pattern of ulcerative colitis.

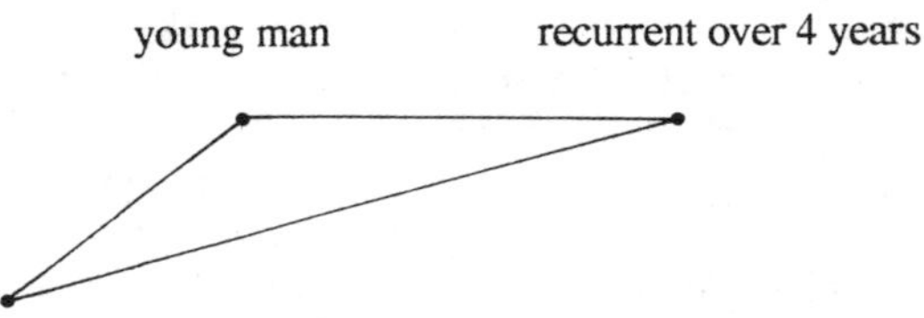

If a third young man has bloody diarrhea after travel to Guatemala, and also numerous previous episodes without travel, which of the points do you connect?

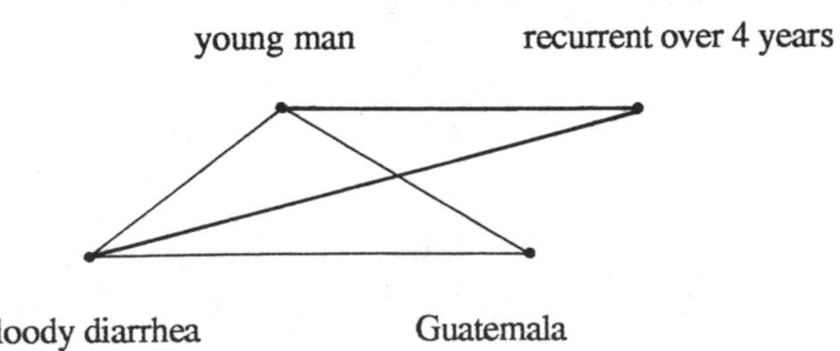

Connecting one set of points makes one figure; connecting a different set makes another. Where one stargazer sees the Big Dipper, another sees the Great Wain, and another the Great Bear. Which you see depends on the points you include and on the pattern you are seeking.

A second problem is that the most salient data points may be buried among other points. If the woman with nausea, fatigue, and secondary amenorrhea also has joint pain, photosensitivity, cough, insomnia, and lymphadenopathy, she may still be pregnant; but it would take a real sleuth to pick out the first three points among the rest. This issue of picking a subset of the data points as the ones to connect makes cluster recognition susceptible to diagnostic prejudice, that is, to looking preferentially for favorite diagnoses.

Finally, cluster recognition is methodless. If you see the pattern, great; if not, there is no way to proceed stepwise toward a goal. Clusters become familiar with experience, but they cannot really be taught.

Method 7. The Systems Approach

The Systems Approach performs differential diagnosis by considering, one at a time, each of the categories of disease mechanism.

1. Genetic/Congenital
2. Mechanical/Traumatic
3. Infectious
4. Neoplastic
5. Immunologic
6. Metabolic
7. Vascular
8. Toxic
9. Degenerative
10. Nutritional

11. Psychogenic
12. Unknown

The actual identities of the categories vary from one author to another, and there is some overlap between them. While some of the labels are self-explanatory, a word of explanation is in order. "Immunologic" embraces the diseases that are predominantly caused by immune mechanisms, including the collagen-vascular disorders, autoimmune diseases, allergy, and immune defects. "Metabolic" diseases include endocrine disorders, many cellular defects, and possibly enzyme deficiencies (some of which are instead categorized as "genetic.") The "Vascular" category embraces disorders caused by thrombosis, vascular insufficiency, and vasculitis (unless the latter is "Immunologic.") "Toxic" disorders are those caused by the chemical action of a foreign substance, including unintended effects of medications. The "Degenerative" category includes disorders characterized by gradual cellular deterioration; examples include Alzheimer's disease and amyotrophic lateral sclerosis (ALS).

Consider the differential diagnosis of diffuse lymphadenopathy in an adolescent.

1. Genetic/Congenital
   - Multicentric eosinophilic granulomatosis
2. Mechanical/Traumatic
   - None
3. Infectious
   - Viral: Epstein-Barr, HIV, hepatitis A, B, C, cytomegalovirus
   - Bacterial: Endocarditis, brucellosis, syphilis
   - Mycobacterial: Tuberculosis
   - Fungal: Histoplasmosis
4. Neoplastic
   - Lymphoma, leukemia
5. Immunologic
   - Systemic lupus, rheumatoid arthritis, sarcoidosis

6. Metabolic
   - None
7. Vascular
   - Vasculitis
8. Toxic
   - None
9. Degenerative
   - None
10. Nutritional
    - None
11. Psychogenic
    - None
12. Unknown
    - Angioimmunoblastic lymphadenopathy

This strategy ensures that you will consider easily overlooked, but important, disease types, such as those in the "Immunologic" or "Congenital" groups. In addition, each category can be divided into subcategories. Thus, considering each infectious agent or syndrome in turn helps you to recall histoplasmosis and syphilis.

The Systems Approach works best for complex, multisystem problems. These are often not localized anatomically and can often arise from diverse mechanisms. Other examples in which this approach may be helpful include peripheral neuropathy, unintended weight loss, night sweats, and multiple organ failure.

The Systems Approach does not work well for acute, localized problems. Fever and pyuria could be due to an infection in the urinary or genital tract, or occasionally to such noninfectious inflammatory states as glomerulonephritis, allergic interstitial nephritis, or interstitial cystitis. It is not much use to go through all the other categories. In addition, the division into categories is a bit messy. It assumes that each disease has a single, known cause; but many diseases involve multiple mechanisms, and in many, the cause is unknown.

SUMMARY

Differential diagnosis by "What Crosses my Mind" or by the "Brilliant Guess," while both common and appealing in some ways, is conceptually bankrupt. The Simple List and the Mnemonic Device are aids to memory, useful and necessary as far as they go, but quite limited. For most clinical problems, the Diagnostic Template is best; its advantages include organizing the diagnostic process along medical concepts, providing entry points for test results, and reusability. Cluster Recognition is compelling, but elusive. Complex medical problems are best tackled either by making multiple diagnostic templates and finding the points of intersection or by the Systems Approach.

CHAPTER 16

Diagnostic Testing

General Principles

1. Differential diagnosis provides an enumeration of the possible. Diagnosis, the target, is concerned less with the possible than with the probable. The purpose of diagnostic testing is to discriminate among diverse diagnostic possibilities and to distinguish the relative probabilities of items on the differential diagnosis.
2. Tests are probability modifiers. They follow a simple design:

Pretest Probability → Test → Posttest Probability

   The *pretest probability* is the likelihood, before performing a particular test, that a patient has a given condition. The *posttest probability* is the likelihood, after performing the test, that the patient has the condition. The results of a test change the probability of the condition under question.
3. Before performing any test, the clinician estimates the pretest probability of the condition under consideration. The pretest probability may be derived from:

- **Prevalence.** The prevalence of cystic fibrosis in the Caucasian American population is known to be about 0.5%. If a new screening test for cystic fibrosis were performed in asymptomatic children, the pretest probability would be 0.5%, or 0.005.
- **Published Studies.** For a number of conditions, studies have been performed that measure the frequency of a given diagnosis in patients with specific clinical findings. For example, a study has reported that in a group of patients with neutropenia and suspected sepsis, the frequency of positive blood cultures was about 10%. One corollary is that, for your patient with neutropenia and suspected sepsis, the pretest probability of bacteremia would be about 10%.
- **Personal Experience.** The clinician estimates, on clinical grounds alone, that the probability of acute appendicitis in a particular young woman with fever, right lower quadrant pain, and diarrhea is about 75%.
- **Educated Guess.** Even if you are not personally familiar with a clinical problem, your background medical knowledge and your reading can lead you toward a ballpark figure. You may never have seen a patient with Jakob-Creutzfeld disease, but you might expect that, in an otherwise healthy, middle-aged man with ataxia and rapidly progressive dementia, the pretest probability might be between 50% and 90%.

4. *The posttest probability always depends on the pretest probability.* This means that a test cannot be interpreted unless you have estimated a pretest probability.
5. In addition, the posttest probability always depends on the operating characteristics of the test.

Test Characteristics

1. A test is defined by two properties: its *sensitivity* and its *specificity*.
2. *Sensitivity* is the probability of a positive test result in a patient with the disease. Sensitivity is also known as the "true-positive rate (TPR)." It is a numeric expression of how well a test correctly identifies patients as having a given disease. In formulaic terms,

$$\text{Sensitivity} = \frac{\text{number of patients with the disease and with a positive test}}{\text{number of patients with the disease}}$$

3. *Specificity* is the probability of a negative test result in a patient without the disease. Specificity is also known as the "true-negative rate (TNR)." It is the numeric expression of how well a test correctly identifies patients as *not* having a given disease. As a formula,

$$\text{Specificity} = \frac{\text{number of patients without the disease and with a negative test}}{\text{number of patients without the disease}}$$

4. The state of being "with a disease" is defined by a *gold standard*, a criterion used to establish the presence or absence of a disease. The ideal gold standard is an indisputable criterion, such as the presence of myocardial necrosis on autopsy. In practice, the gold standards are often imperfect; a surrogate gold standard in coronary artery disease is the coronary angiogram.
5. A test is characterized by comparing it with a gold standard. This comparison is effected by a standard format, the 2 × 2 Table:

	Gold-Std positive	Gold-Std negative
Test positive		
Test negative		

6. A given test result falls into four possible categories, when compared with the gold standard:

   True positive: Gold-standard positive, test positive

   True negative: Gold-standard negative, test negative

   False positive: Gold-standard negative, test positive

   False negative: Gold-standard positive, test negative

	Gold-Std positive	Gold-Std negative	
Test positive	true positives (TP)	false positives (FP)	Total with pos test
			+
Test negative	false negatives (FN)	true negatives (TN)	Total with
	Total with disease +	Total without disease	= N

N refers to the total number of patients in the study population.

7. These values are often depicted like this:

	Gold-Std positive	Gold-Std negative	
Test positive	a	b	a + b
Test negative	c	d	c + d
	a + c	b + d	N

Thus, on a 2 × 2 table,

$$\text{Sensitivity} = a/(a + c)$$
$$\text{Specificity} = d/(b + d)$$

OR

$$\text{Sensitivity} = TP/(TP + FN)$$
$$\text{Specificity} = TN/(FP + TN)$$

Using Tests

1. Sensitivity and specificity refer to the test alone, independent of any application. What the clinician wants to know is, "What does a positive or negative test result tell me about my patient?" This is the posttest probability, or *posterior probability*.
2. The posttest probability of a positive test, coded as

PTP(+), is the likelihood that a patient has a given disease if the test is positive. Referring to the 2 × 2 Table,

$$\begin{aligned} PTP(+) &= a/(a+b) \\ &= TP/(TP+FP) \end{aligned}$$

3. The posttest probability of a negative test, coded as PTP(−), is the likelihood that a patient has a given disease if the test is negative. On the 2 × 2 Table,

$$\begin{aligned} PTP(-) &= c/(c+d) \\ &= FN/(FN+TN) \end{aligned}$$

4. Two terms related to PTP(+) and PTP(−) are the *positive predictive value* (PPV) and the *negative predictive value* (NPV). The PPV refers to a study population and is the proportion of patients with a positive test result who have the disease. The NPV, again referring to a study population, is the proportion of patients with a negative test result who do not have the disease. PPV is sometimes used interchangeably with PTP(+). Note, however, that PTP(+) depends on the pretest probability whatever the circumstances, while the PPV depends on prevalence. Thus, PPV is a special case of PTP(+). A word of caution: NPV is not interchangeable with PTP(−). PTP(−) is the probability of disease, given a negative test. NPV is the probability of no disease, given a negative test. PTP(−) is thus comparable to 1−NPV.

5. It warrants repetition: The posttest probability always depends on the pretest probability.

Example: *The Flicker Test*

An ophthalmologist has recommended a new test for detecting glaucoma, the Flicker test. You want to decide whether to refer your patients for the test.

In the principal study of the Flicker test, the test was performed on 1000 persons. Intraocular pressure (IOP) was also measured by Schiotz's tonometry in each person. Intraocular hypertension was defined as IOP >21 mm Hg.

Data:

IOP by tonometry was >21 mm in 100 persons and ≤21 mm in 900.

Flicker test was positive in 75 persons with IOP >21 mm.

Flicker test was negative in 720 persons with IOP ≤21 mm.

Procedure:

First, make a 2 × 2 table.

	IOP >21 mm	**IOP ≤21 mm**	
Flicker Test positive	75		
Flicker Test negative		720	
	100	900	1000

Then, complete the Table by simple arithmetic.

	IOP >21 mm	**IOP ≤21 mm**	
Flicker Test positive	75	180	255
Flicker Test negative	25	720	745
	100	900	1000

Calculate sensitivity and specificity.

$$\begin{aligned} \text{Sensitivity} &= a/(a + c) \\ &= 75/100 \\ &= 75\% \text{ (OR: 0.75)} \\ \text{Specificity} &= d/(b + d) \\ &= 720/900 \\ &= 80\% \text{ (OR: 0.80)} \end{aligned}$$

Calculate PTP.

$$\begin{aligned} \text{PTP}(+) &= a/(a + b) \\ &= 75/255 \\ &= 33.3\% \\ \text{PTP}(-) &= c/(c + d) \\ &= 25/745 \\ &= 3.4\% \end{aligned}$$

Interpret.

A positive test means that the patient has a 33.3% probability of having intraocular hypertension.

A negative test means that the patient has a 3.4% probability of having intraocular hypertension.

6. Understanding how this works will allow you to order tests and interpret them wisely. *Most people, including most doctors, do not understand this.* They think that a positive test means that the patient has the disease, and that a negative test means that the patient does not have the disease. In fact, in this example, the patient with a positive test has only a one-third probability of disease.
7. *Bayes' theorem* is an algebraic formulation of the 2 × 2 Table. To calculate PTP(+) using Bayes' theorem, you need to know:
   - The sensitivity of the test (TPR)
   - The FPR

   FPR = proportion of persons without disease who have positive test
   = b/(b + d)

- The pretest probability = pD

Using this information,

$$\text{PTP}(+) = \frac{\text{pD} \times \text{TPR}}{(\text{pD} \times \text{TPR}) + [(1 - \text{pD}) \times \text{FPR}]}$$

Bayes' theorem may be attractive to the mathematically minded, but it has no other advantage over the 2 × 2 Table. Its disadvantage is that it covers over the significance of the terms.

Choosing Tests

1. The ideal test is 100% sensitive and 100% specific. The only trouble is that no such test exists.
2. Lesser sensitivities and specificities are accepted according to the type of information that is needed. If missing the diagnosis would be disastrous, choose a test with the best sensitivity. For example, the diagnosis of subarachnoid hemorrhage can be made by CT scan or by lumbar puncture. CT is less traumatic and is usually performed first. Lumbar puncture is more sensitive, though less specific. If you need to be certain regarding hemorrhage, lumbar puncture should be performed even if the CT does not show bleeding.

   If, on the other hand, frequent false positives would be problematic, choose a test that has a high specificity. For example, thermography is a radiographic technique that achieved some popularity for detecting breast cancer. But because the specificity of the test was only 70%, many women were told erroneously that they may have breast cancer, leading to unnecessary worry and procedures.
3. Choose a test that maximizes the difference between the pretest probability and the posttest probability. A good test would be one for which a positive result increased the probability of disease greatly and a negative result decreased the probabil-

ity of disease greatly. This relation can be depicted as follows:

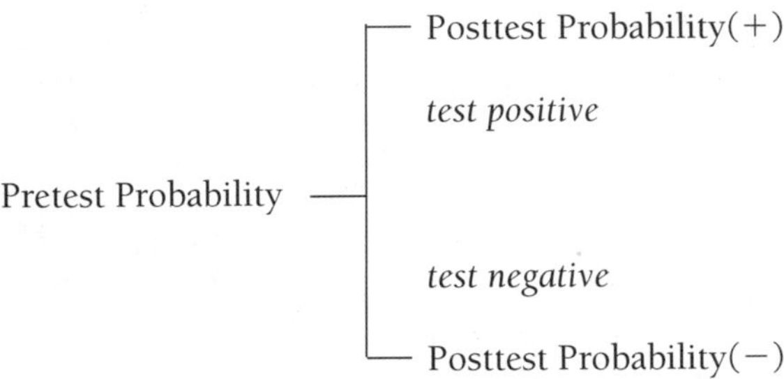

In the example of the Flicker test, for a pretest probability of 10%, the posttest probability after a positive test is 33%, and the posttest probability after a negative test is 3%.

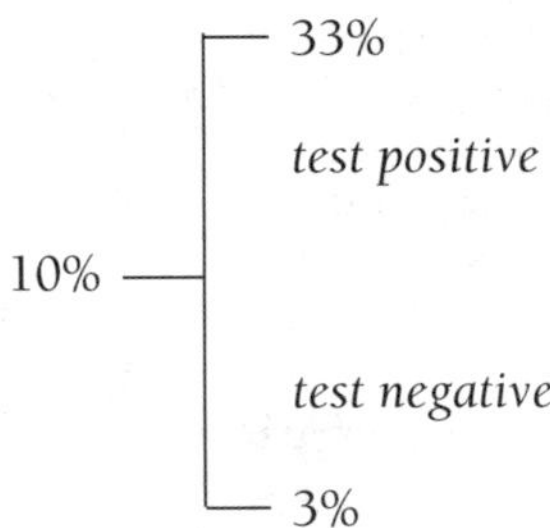

The splay, then, of the Flicker test, is fairly good.

4. Other reasons to prefer Test A to Test B include:
   - Test A involves less risk.
   - Test A is less expensive.
   - Test A confers a higher degree of certainty.
   - Test A has a greater splay, as described above.
   - Test A is more readily available.
   - You have more experience with Test A.
   - The patient finds Test A more acceptable or congenial.

Continuous Values

1. Not all tests give results that are simply "positive" or "negative." While the 2 × 2 Table implies a binary system of test results, many test results give continuous values. For example, an AST level is expressed as a number ranging from 0 to 5000 U/L or greater, not simply as "elevated" or "not elevated."
2. How are different degress of abnormality interpreted?
   - In general, the greater the deviation from normal, the more likely that a positive test result is a true positive. A patient with AST 1000 U/L is more likely to have acute hepatitis than a patient with AST 100 U/L.
   - In general, the greater the deviation from normal, the more severe the disease is likely to be. A patient with AST 1000 U/L is likely to have more severe hepatitis than the patient with AST 100 U/L.
3. **Cut-Off Analysis.** To convert a continuous variable to a binary "positive or negative" result, a cut-off point is selected. The cut-off point is a value for the test result used to define positive and negative results. Test results on one side of the cut-off point are defined as positive, and results on the other side are defined as negative. In the glaucoma example, intraocular pressure of 21 mm Hg was chosen as the cut-off value.

   The choice of the cut-off point has a major effect on the meaning of a test result. If the cut-off point is chosen near the extreme of a distribution, the test will be specific but not sensitive. If the cut-off point is chosen near the median of a distribution, the test will be sensitive but not specific.

   In general, for a given test, adjustments that improve sensitivity tend to decrease specificity, and vice versa. For example, significant depression of the ST segment on the EKG is defined to be 1 mV or greater. If the cut-off point were reset to be

0.5 mV, the test would capture more persons with angina; it would be more sensitive. On the other hand, the test would also capture more persons who did not have angina; it would be less specific. A test that is too sensitive is like a car alarm that goes off any time a bus passes.

Combining Tests

1. The probability of two *independent* events is the product of the probabilities of each event. If two tests were completely independent, then the posttest probability [PTP(+)] after Test A and Test B would be PTP(+) A × PTP(+) B.
2. In clinical medicine, tests related to a single condition are usually not independent of each other.
3. Since tests are usually performed sequentially, the posttest probability of the earlier test becomes the pretest probability of the later test.

Screening Tests

1. *Diagnostic tests* are usually employed to identify conditions for which positive evidence is apparent. Examples include the Pap smear in a woman with vaginal bleeding or syphilis serology in a man with anterior uveitis. The main purposes of diagnostic tests, considered in this sense, are:
   - To assess a diagnostic hypothesis
   - To confirm or to refute a proposed diagnosis

   This second sense, sometimes called "ruling in" or "ruling out," warrants caution. A diagnosis is confirmed only when a gold-standard definition is met, for example by a biopsy. A diagnosis is excluded only when some finding is incompatible with the diagnosis; for example, a normal lumbar puncture excludes the possibility of acute meningitis. These absolute conditions, which imply probabilities of

100% or 0%, are not usually met in clinical medicine. Be careful: a normal EKG does not rule out an acute MI; a normal chest radiograph does not rule out pneumonia; and a negative antinuclear antibody does not rule out systemic lupus.

2. *Screening tests* are those used to identify problems for which no positive evidence is apparent. Examples include the Pap smear in asymptomatic women or a syphilis serology in routine marriage applications. There are three main purposes for screening tests:
   - Early detection of disease
   - Identification of risk factors
   - "Completing the data base"—controversial. An example is the chest x-ray on hospital admission before elective cholecystectomy. If there is no reason to suspect that the patient has cardiac or pulmonary disease, the physician orders a chest x-ray in the belief that its findings need to be known, in the interest of completeness. Note that most apparently healthy persons who undergo elective surgery will have normal chest x-rays, and that the decision involves an extra $80 to $150 for every operation.
3. A screening test is applied to the general population when a condition is prevalent throughout the public at large. An example includes BP measurement. A screening test is applied to a select population when the condition is especially prevalent in a particular group. The PPD (purified protein derivative) skin test for tuberculosis is performed occasionally in the general public but annually in health care workers, a group at increased risk of tuberculosis.
4. The ideal screening test meets several criteria. There should be a "burden of suffering:" that is, the disease being tested for should be fairly common in the population at hand, and the disease should

cause significant morbidity or mortality. The disease should be detectable at an early, treatable, presymptomatic stage. Screening smokers for lung cancer with chest x-rays can detect cancer, but not at a treatable stage; it is therefore not recommended. Early intervention should be able to affect the outcome. Mammography is an effective screening test because breast cancers are curable in an early stage but fatal in an advanced stage. A screening test should have low cost, low discomfort, and low risk. Finally, it should have a high specificity; that is, there should be a low proportion of false positives. In screening for colon cancer with stool guaiac cards, a false positive generally means an unnecessary colonoscopy, with attendant cost, inconvenience, and risk.

5. The pretest probability of a screening test is the prevalence of the condition in the population being studied.

CHAPTER 17

Diagnosis

General Principles

1. The term *diagnosis* is used in two different ways. In the simplest sense, diagnosis is the name given to a medical condition. Diagnosis also refers to the process of arriving at this name.
2. A diagnosis carries the sense of a discrete, well-defined, pathophysiologic entity. Thus, *rash* is not a diagnosis; rash can refer to a variety of different conditions. *Headache* is not a diagnosis, but *tension headache*, *migraine*, and *cluster headache* are diagnoses.
3. The names given in diagnosis are the names of diseases and syndromes. A *disease* is a characteristic, well-defined, consistent pattern of body dysfunction. Examples include renal cell carcinoma, measles, and sclerosing cholangitis. A *syndrome* is a pattern of clinical findings. Examples include Down syndrome, Felty's syndrome, and Reiter's syndrome. Historically, when a new state of unwellness is first recognized, it takes shape as a pattern of findings, a syndrome. Later, when the condition is better characterized and understood, it graduates to the status of a disease. However, the label of "syndrome" often sticks even when the condition is well understood. Down syndrome is every bit as well understood as sclerosing cholangitis, yet it is still called a syndrome. Thus, the

distinction between a disease and a syndrome is considerably blurred.

Disease and syndrome should both be distinguished from *illness*, which is the patient's subjective experience of unwellness. An illness is the manifestation of a disease in an individual patient.

4. In our era, a diagnosis also carries the sense of a plausible pathophysiologic mechanism. The 5q– syndrome, a form of myelodysplasia, functions as a diagnosis in part because the deletion of the long arm of chromosome 5 might be credibly linked to hematologic disregulation.
5. *Accurate diagnosis is the keystone of modern medical therapy.* Not all medical systems are based on diagnosis: neither ancient Chinese medicine, nor traditional Navajo medicine, nor Western medicine before the 19th century places it centrally. *In our medical system, however, a specific diagnosis is crucial, because it leads to a specific treatment.*
6. *General therapy*, also called "supportive" or "symptomatic therapy," is medical treatment that tends to help in an inexact way. General therapy may be directed toward relief of symptoms, such as an analgesic, or to support of overall recuperation, such as rest. General therapies are used for a broad variety of disorders. Acetaminophen, for example, is a good antipyretic for any cause of fever. *Specific therapy* is treatment that works for a specific diagnosis. Penicillin works for pneumonia caused by Pneumococcus and a few other organisms; it does not work for other pneumonias, and it does not help cough caused by noninfectious mechanisms. Specific therapies rarely provide immediate symptom relief, except to the extent that they treat the underlying cause of the symptom.
7. Consider a child with sore throat and fever. Until 1748, the child would receive a diagnosis of

pharyngitis. Treatment would be supportive; for example, gargles and the like. In that year, an English physician named John Fothergill accurately described the specific form of sore throat that was later called "diphtheria," a new clinical entity.

In 1883, the diphtheria organism was discovered. Acknowledging the infectious nature of diphtheria, physicians treated all children suspected of having diphtheria with quarantine and fumigation. Admittedly, many of these children did not have diphtheria, and the treatment was not terribly effective, but something was being done.

In 1892, a test for the diphtheria organism was developed. Thus, the physician could now tell whether or not the patient had diphtheria. Children who had a positive test were treated with quarantine and fumigation. Children with a negative test received supportive measures, and they were no longer endangered by quarantine with test-positive patients.

In 1891, a specific treatment, antitoxin, first appeared. Antitoxin worked for children with diphtheria and was often life-saving. Antitoxin was not beneficial for children without diphtheria—and it was a rather uncomfortable and expensive treatment. Children who had a positive test for diphtheria therefore received antitoxin; children with a negative test again received supportive measures.

This scene from recent medical history illustrates a crucial point: the diagnosis matters, because it leads to a specific treatment that works. The point is not obvious, although we often take it for granted. If a child is shown to have diphtheria, a life-saving treatment is at hand. It is thus imperative to know if the child has diphtheria or not. If a patient has chest pain, it is imperative that the clinician determine whether the correct diagnosis is acute MI, aortic dissection, pulmonary embolism, or some other cause. Each of these diagnoses responds to therapy, but each responds to a specific therapy for that diagnosis. A wrong diagnosis means a wrong treatment, which may end in catastrophe.

8. There are two additional reasons to pursue a diagnosis. One relates to the power of naming. An internist of my acquaintance was assigned, while in the military, to serve as the base dermatologist, despite his scanty knowledge of that subspecialty. He developed the strategy of describing whatever skin lesions he observed and translating the description into Latin. Thus, a patient with little red spots was given a diagnosis of maculae rubrae parvae—and the patient was satisfied, having received no more than a name. Even when no treatment is available, a diagnosis gives patients the sense that their conditions are known and manageable—and also that their physician is knowledgeable and empowered. This helps to activate the healing process.
9. An additional advantage of diagnosis is its role in prognosis. *Prognosis* is the prediction of the likely course of a disease. If a definitive diagnosis can be given, the future course of the illness can be foreseen to some degree. This provides the patient with invaluable information, including the probability of recovery, deterioration, or death. Prognosis was central to Hippocratic medicine and was the basis for the school's emphasis on diagnosis, even when effective treatment was not at hand.
10. *Differential diagnosis* provides a list of possible hypotheses. *Diagnostic testing* modifies the relative probabilities of these hypotheses. Diagnosis chooses among the possible hypotheses. If differential diagnosis results in a kind of nomination,

diagnostic testing is a primary election, and diagnosis is the election.

When diagnostic testing is complete, the clinician has a list of possible diagnoses with their relative probabilities. The next step is to choose one of these hypotheses to act on. There are several criteria for this selection.

- **Prevalence.** Prevalence might refer to:
  - The frequency of a condition in the overall population.
  - The frequency of a condition in the type of patient at hand—you imagine a population subgroup whose members resemble your patient.

  Remember too that in outbreaks or epidemics, the prevalence of a disease can increase abruptly.
- **Coherence.** Does the diagnosis fit pathophysio logic reasoning?
- **Completeness.** Does the diagnosis fit as much of the clinical scenario as possible?
- **Economy: Occam's famous razor.** Can a small number of hypotheses be invoked to explain the disease?
- Maxim: "Atypical presentations of common diseases occur more frequently than typical presentations of uncommon diseases." For example, a patient with pain in the right middle abdomen is more likely to have appendicitis with an unusual pain localization than a Meckel's diverticulum.
- Does the diagnosis capture the essence of the illness, the central problem? A disease has primary, secondary, and subsidiary findings; diagnosis must discriminate between these and focus on primary findings. A diagnosis that accounts for all of the features of an illness is called a *unifying diagnosis*; the unifying diagnosis is often not apparent until some time has passed.

Diagnosis and Decision

1. Diagnosis is not an end in itself. The primary reason to attain a diagnosis is to provide a treatment.
2. Diagnosis thus brings two imperatives into conflict: the desire to know and the desire to act. If certainty in diagnosis were the only goal, the physician could think about and perform diagnostic tests indefinitely. However, the lengthy process needed to achieve certainty may not be desirable if:
   - Early treatment is desirable.

     > ***Example:*** Heparin is often started for patients with suspected pulmonary embolism even before a pulmonary angiogram or ventilation-perfusion scan is performed.

   - The disease is minor or self-limiting.

     > ***Example:*** If a patient has a routine upper respiratory syndrome, it is not necessary to perform serologic tests to determine exactly which virus is present.

   - The cost of further testing—as measured in dollars, patient discomfort, or delay—is not justified by the situation at hand.
3. As the diagnostic process proceeds in time, the probability of a given diagnosis increases. If the patient is untreated during this time, however, delay, cost, and risk are accruing. *Thus, for every condition, there is a point at which the probability of a given diagnosis is sufficiently high to warrant treatment.* This point is called the *threshold.*
4. *The degree of certainty needed to institute treatment varies according to the diagnosis being considered.* In a patient with leukopenia and fever, prompt treatment for possible bacteremia is usually started even if the probability of bacteremia is low. Broad-spec-

trum intravenous antibiotics are administered because the risk of bacteremia, if untreated, in these patients is so high. On the other hand, in a patient with suspected leukemia, bone marrow biopsy is always performed before instituting anti-leukemia therapy, even if the probability of acute leukemia is high. Certainty in diagnosis is mandatory because the risks of the drugs used to treat leukemia are so high. In a patient with suspected MI but nondiagnostic EKG changes, sublingual nitroglycerin is administered early, because it has a low risk of toxicity. Thrombolytic agents are usually not administered in this setting, because they carry a relatively high risk of significant toxicity.

5. A few guidelines apply.
   - The more beneficial early treatment, the lower the threshold for treating.
   - The more toxic the treatment, the higher the threshold for treating.
   - The more serious the disease, the higher the need for certain diagnosis.
6. For purposes of treatment, identifying the class of disorders to which a disease belongs may be nearly as good as achieving a definitive diagnosis. In a patient with 3 months of symmetric polyarthritis, synovial thickening, morning stiffness, anemia, fever, and an elevated sedimentation rate, it may be adequate to decide that the patient has an apparent collagen-vascular disorder and to begin treatment, even if the rheumatologic serologies are not diagnostic. This decision is aided by the fact that treatments are often specific for a class of disorders rather than for individual diagnoses only. Glucocorticoids are an effective treatment for many of the collagen-vascular disorders, whether systemic lupus or rheumatoid arthritis or another of the class.
7. The threshold at which a given action is indicated can be modeled mathematically by *Decision Analy-*

sis. Decision Analysis is a formal technique for quantifying decisions by assigning relative values to the possible outcomes of a choice. Decision Analysis is at present too cumbersome for use in individual patients, but it is a useful construct for considering clinical decisions for large numbers of patients in certain scenarios.

8. Every book needs a joke; this one carries the dignity and the shop-worn raggedness of time. Four physicians go duck hunting: a neurologist, an internist, a surgeon, and a pathologist. They are sitting side by side in the swamp, guns across their knees, when a bird shape flies overhead.

   Neurologist: "It's a duck." [returns to his reading].

   Internist: "It looks like a duck . . . of course it could be a goose, and it might be a crane; a turkey is possible, and I can't rule out a pterodactyl. . ."

   Surgeon: "A duck!" [pulls out a howitzer and blasts it into the air. A mess of flesh and feathers drifts downward.]

   Pathologist: [toeing the carcass] "It was a duck."

Problems in Diagnosis

1. Diagnoses are names, but they consist of diverse sorts of names. A diagnosis might be named for:
   - A pathologic finding, such as MI or a glioblastoma. Most diseases are named or defined in this way.
   - An abnormal state, such as thrombocytopenia or thyrotoxicosis.
   - An abnormal process, such as transient ischemic attack.
   - An effect implied by a cause, such as cyanide poisoning.
   - A propensity, such as irritable bowel disease.

2. Diagnosis requires a match between disparate systems of understanding disease. One match is encapsulated in the distinction between illness and disease: the physician must match the patient's subjective experience of unwellness with a biomedical conception of disease. This frequently creates tension between the patient and the physician. The patient may feel that the physician is trying to fit the illness to a stereotypical pattern, destroying its individuality. The physician, meanwhile, may feel that the patient is resisting diagnosis by failing to present a classic picture found in the textbooks of medicine.
3. At the same time, the clinician must match clinical observations to what the pathologist might see, were tissue to be examined. Most diseases, in our era, are defined in terms of pathologic and histologic findings. However, the physician often renders a diagnosis without examining tissue specimens. A patient who has acute chest pain, ST-segment elevations on EKG, and positive creatine kinase MB enzymes is said to be having an MI, even though no myocardial biopsy is performed. The physician infers the presence of infarction—a histologic finding—from the clinical picture.
4. There are other problems with histologic-based diagnosis. Histology describes an end state, not the process of arriving there. For example, it can show an atherosclerotic plaque in a carotid artery and an infarction of the cerebral cortex but not the hypercholesterolemia, tobacco use, and arterial hypertension that led to these outcomes. Histology misses the dynamic features of an illness; it can demonstrate a thyroid nodule but not thyrotoxicosis, mitral stenosis but not atrial fibrillation, pyelonephritis but not sepsis. Further, the presence of an abnormal histologic finding may not mean *clinically* important disease. If the prevalence of

prostate cancer in 90-year-old men approaches 100%, what is the significance of a prostate biopsy that shows a few carcinoma cells? Does the man have prostate cancer, in the sense that we conceive it? Should anything be done about it?

5. Diagnosis is beleaguered with problems in probabilistic thinking. Clinical language often clouds quantitative probabilities with terms such as "suggestive of," "consistent with," "cannot rule out." These may be necessary, but they are quite imprecise. Whatever the patient actually has, no matter how rare, has a probability in *him or her* of 100%. People do contract rare diseases—rarely—and these need to be considered.
6. Premises regarding normality and variation underlie much of diagnostic thinking. While we are all familiar with the normal distribution illustrated by the bell-shaped curve, many clinical phenomena—for instance, blood pressure—follow other distributions. The decision whether a finding is abnormal, or a normal variation, can be vexing: consider left-handedness, or freckles, or Gilbert syndrome. Larger deviations from normal values are usually significant, indicating both a higher probability of abnormality and a higher degree of abnormality. Smaller deviations may or may not be significant. A palpable spleen tip in an adult, no matter how slight, is probably important, while a platelet count of 140,000/μL (normal 150,000 to 400,000/μL) is probably not.
7. A diagnosis should be considered a working hypothesis and a basis for action. The clinician must often accept some measure of uncertainty in order to act promptly. At the same time, he or she must remain open-minded to alternative diagnoses. One of the greatest pitfalls in clinical thinking is the tendency to reject data that contradict a favored diag-

nosis. One should search for alternative diagnoses when:

- The patient isn't getting better.
- The disease isn't following the expected pattern.
- New data, or old data newly considered, do not fit the working diagnosis.

CHAPTER 18

Clinical Case Problems

Approach to Solving Clinical Cases

Each case is designed to illustrate a step in the diagnostic process. You should focus your attention on this step.

The sequence for solving the cases is the one outlined in Chapters 14 to 17:

1. Problem list
2. Differential diagnosis
3. Diagnostic testing
4. Diagnosis
5. Treatment

Instructions:

1. Read the case.
2. Read through the questions and answer them.
3. Then consult the answers, given on the next page. You will learn more if you do not consult the answers until you have grappled with solving the problems on your own.

The cases and names are true, ". . . mainly. There was things which he stretched, but mainly he told the truth."[1]

[1]Mark Twain: The Adventures of Huckleberry Finn.

CASE 1

Wilma Trager

Wilma Trager is a 52-year-old woman who consults you in the outpatient clinic because she feels dizzy. She says that she has had occasional headaches for many years but felt well otherwise until 2 weeks ago, when she began to note upper abdominal pain. The pain was described as a "burning" feeling above the umbilicus, worst in the morning, relieved by food, and somewhat increased in severity in the last 3 days. Today, she woke with the usual pain but felt "dizzy, like I was going to faint," without vertigo, when she stood up; symptoms resolved after she lay down for a few minutes.

The Past Medical History is otherwise unremarkable. She takes ibuprofen 400 mg every 6 to 8 hours and has no known drug allergies. She smokes one pack of cigarettes daily and drinks 2 to 4 glasses of zinfandel per night on weekends. She works as a twisting supervisor in a pretzel bakery and is married with two children.

1. At this point, make a problem list based on the history.

On physical examination, the patient looked slightly pale but generally well. Vital signs: Temp 37.2° orally, BP 130/84 supine, 110/68 erect; HR 92 supine, 112 erect. Notable findings included mild tenderness in the epigastric area and black stool that was guaiac-positive for heme.

2. At this point, make a problem list based on the physical exam.

3. Now, make a prioritized list based on the history and physical, ranking the problems from most important to least important.

Answers for Case 1

1. Problem list from history

Dizzy
Headaches
Abdominal pain
Ibuprofen use
Smoking
Alcohol (zinfandel) use
? Demanding lifestyle

2. Problem list from physical exam

Orthostatic hypotension
Epigastric tenderness
Guaiac-positive stool; could also be coded as GI bleeding

3. Prioritized problem list from history and exam

a. Orthostatic hypotension (first because it implies an acute hemorrhage of substantial quantity and is therefore the most life-threatening).
b. Guaiac-positive stool/GI bleed (could be first if considered as the most basic problem, the essence of the case).
c. Light-headedness (subsidiary here to orthostatic hypotension, since it's part of the same problem). Note that the chief complaint is not necessarily the first problem.
d. Abdominal pain.
e. Ibuprofen use.
f. Smoking.
g. Alcohol.
h. Headaches.
i. ? Demanding lifestyle, ? depression/anxiety.

Tips

1. Identify the problems. A problem may be a symptom, a sign, or physical finding, a habit, a psychosocial element, or any other clue. It should be noteworthy but need not be abnormal.
2. Problems can be dealt with more easily if the patient's description is translated into clinical language (e.g., dizziness : light-headedness).
3. **Lumping and splitting.** Orthostatic hypotension, dizziness, and light-headedness are all part of a single problem. GI bleed should not be lumped together with these, for the present. Although GI bleed is the likely cause for these findings, lumping them together at this point is premature and makes too strong an assumption about the pathophysiology.
4. In ranking problems, greater priority is given to:
   - Life-threatening conditions
   - Acute conditions
   - Fixable conditions: Wherever interceding is most important
   - "Hard data" (GI bleed is hard; headache here is soft.)
5. Note that the problem list defines the field of inquiry. Research in clinical reasoning has shown that skilled diagnosticians are distinguished from amateurs by the way they frame the problem at hand. Embarking on an investigation of "dizziness" would miss the mark.

CASE 2

Stetson SanSouci

Stetson SanSouci is a 26-year-old saxophone player who comes to the Emergency Room because of fever and cough for 2 days. He says that he felt well until 1 week ago, when he developed "cold" symptoms consisting of sore throat, runny nose, and sneezing. These improved over the next several days until 2 days ago, when he developed fever to 102°F, cough productive of brown sputum, and discomfort in the right side of the chest that was increased with deep breath or cough. Symptoms continued despite a topical liniment. On the day of admission, he noticed dyspnea while climbing stairs and decided to come to the hospital.

The Past Medical History is unremarkable. He takes no medicines but is allergic to penicillin, which caused hives in childhood. He does not smoke, and he drinks 1 to 2 glasses of wine per night on weekends. He is single, keeps both a parakeet and a tarantula, and denies HIV risk factors.

On Physical Examination, the patient looks well-developed but moderately ill. Vital signs: Temperature 38.6°C orally, BP 170/102, HR 100, RR 22. Notable findings include mild oropharyngeal erythema, coarse breath sounds with egophony in the right midfield, and a 3-cm flat pigmented lesion on the left lateral thigh.

1. Make a problem list based on the history and physical.

2. Now re-rank the problems based on their relative importance.

3. What is the best way to combine and separate the problems?

Answers for Case 2

1. Problem list from history and physical

Fever
Cough
Recent "cold"
Brown sputum
Pleuritic chest pain (note the translation)
Dyspnea
Penicillin allergy
Parakeet (not tarantula; while a parakeet raises the question of psittacosis, the tarantula is irrelevant)
Looks acutely ill
Elevated BP
Tachypnea
Oropharyngeal edema
Rhonchi
Egophony
Pigmented lesion

2. Prioritized list

a. Pulmonary findings
   - Productive cough (here lumping cough and brown sputum)
   - Dyspnea/tachypnea
   - Rhonchi
   - Egophony

b. Looks ill/fever
c. Pigmented lesion
d. Parakeet
e. Recent upper respiratory symptoms, oropharyngeal erythema
f. Elevated BP
g. Tachycardia
h. Penicillin allergy

3. Lumping and splitting

As grouped above

Tips

1. An additional principle in ranking problems is the type of significance a piece of data may potentially carry. The parakeet is potentially significant because of psittacosis, a form of pneumonia that is transmitted by these birds and by parrots. The tarantula can bite but is irrelevant to the syndrome at hand.
2. Data that can be readily subsumed under another problem are demoted in priority. Tachycardia in a person with pneumonia does not carry much information value. It would be notable in a healthy young man at rest.
3. Time considerations also affect the way problems are ranked. Note the different temporal features of the problems in this case.
   - Active now and urgent: Pneumonia
   - Active now but not urgent: Hypertension
   - Present now but readily explained by the situation: Tachycardia
   - Present but unrelated to the problem at hand: Pigmented lesion
4. A drug allergy should always be listed as a problem. However, its priority is rather low, unless there are so many allergies that few antibiotic choices remain.
5. Alcohol consumption, if modest, need not be listed as a problem—unless a condition is present, such as chronic pancreatitis, that makes any alcohol consumption deleterious.

CASE 3

Keebler Nobbit

Keebler Nobbit is a 56-year-old man who comes to your office because of nausea for 3 weeks. He has always felt well and was told at an annual check-up with another doctor 10 months ago that everything was normal. Nausea began 3 weeks ago, without any clear provocation, and has waxed and waned since. It does not vary with food or position. There is no headache and no abdominal pain.

The Past Medical History is unremarkable. He takes no medicines, has no known drug allergies, smokes one pack of cigarettes daily and drinks one to two beers a month. He works as a helicopter pilot and is divorced with two children.

On Physical Exam, the patient looks icteric but is in no distress. Vital signs: Temp 36.8°C orally, BP 122/84, HR 88. Notable findings include icterus of the sclera, buccal mucosa, and skin. There is mild tenderness in the right periumbilical area.

1. Make a problem list based on the history and physical.

2. Write out a template for his jaundice.

You decide to order blood tests. Findings include:

CBC normal
Reticulocyte count normal
Electrolytes normal
SGOT and SGPT normal
LDH normal

Alkaline phosphatase 240	(normal 30 to 110 U/L)
Direct bilirubin 4.2	(normal 0.1 to 0.3 mg/dL)
Indirect bilirubin 0.7	(normal 0.1 to 0.7 mg/dL)

3. How do the lab data help to locate the patient's jaundice on the diagnostic template?

4. What is the likely cause of this patient's jaundice?

Answers for Case 3

1. Problem list for the history and exam

Jaundice or icterus
Nausea
Tenderness in the right periumbilical area

2. Diagnostic template for jaundice

Note that this template can be reused for any case involving jaundice.

Items in italics are more detailed than necessary for the present exercise.

- I. Indirect hyperbilirubinemia
  - A. Increased bili production
    - 1. Hemolysis
    - 2. *Ineffective erythropoiesis*
  - B. Decreased bili uptake (*Flavaspidic acid, used to treat tapeworm; some Gilbert*)
  - C. Decreased bili conjugation (*Gilbert, Crigler-Najjar*)
- II. Direct hyperbilirubinemia
  - A. Intrahepatic cholestasis
    - 1. Decreased excretion of normal bili conjugates
      - a. Due to hepatocyte damage
        - (1) Infection
        - (2) Toxin (alcohol, drug, mushroom, chemicals)
        - (3) Severe systemic illness (shock, sepsis, etc.)
        - (4) *Budd-Chiari*
        - (5) *Acute fatty liver of pregnancy*
      - b. Without hepatocyte damage
        - (1) Congenital (*Dubin-Johnson, Rotor's*)
        - (2) Acquired
          - (a) Drug

(b) Toxin
(c) *Severe systemic illness*
(d) *Primary biliary cirrhosis*
(e) Pregnancy

B. Extrahepatic cholestasis
   1. Extrinsic compression: Mass lesion
   2. Intrinsic obstruction
      a. Stone
      b. Stricture
      c. Tumor
      d. *Sclerosing cholangitis*

3. Using lab data to locate a case within the template

The principal bilirubin pattern is direct hyperbilirubinemia.

The principal liver-test pattern implies cholestasis. Hepatocyte damage is not evident.

4. Likely cause of the patient's jaundice

The laboratory tests leave us with three categories:

Cholestasis Without Hepatocyte Damage. But there is no history of drug or toxin, and no sign of a severe systemic illness. The bilirubin is rather high for congenital processes. Primary biliary cirrhosis should have a very high alkaline phosphatase before jaundice sets in.

Extrinsic Compression of the Biliary Tree. Fits all the data.

Intrinsic Obstruction of the Biliary Tree. The history does not fit cholelithiasis. Stricture, biliary carcinoma and sclerosing cholangitis are possible but less common than a mass lesion of the pancreas.

The most likely diagnosis is extrinsic compression of the common bile duct due to cancer of the head of the pancreas. A sonogram or CT scan would confirm this impression.

Tips

1. In applying the diagnostic template, the first step is to see whether the pattern of bilirubin elevation is primarily indirect or direct.
   - *For indirect hyperbilirubinemia:*
     - If the reticulocyte count and LDH are elevated, hemolysis is likely to be present. Haptoglobin should be decreased, and the Coombs' test is often positive.
     - If the reticulocyte count is normal but LDH is elevated, ineffective erythropoiesis is likely.
     - If both the reticulocyte count and LDH are normal, decreased bilirubin uptake or conjugation is likely.
   - For direct hyperbilirubinemia:
     - If the predominant liver test abnormality is an increase in SGOT and SGPT, hepatocyte damage is likely.
     - If the predominant liver test abnormality is a predominance of alkaline phosphatase, cholestasis is likely.
     - Within these categories, types are distinguished on clinical grounds.
2. Subsequent reasoning depends on comparing the possible diagnoses to the clinical scenario and evaluating for the "best fit."

CASE 4

Dottie Dieffendorfer

Dottie Dieffendorfer is a 28-year-old woman who comes to your office because of itching for 3 weeks. She first noted itching 3 weeks ago, involving first the left kneecap and then the entire body. Over-the-counter medications have not helped. She feels well otherwise and has had no medical problems in the past. Medicines include calamine lotion, diphenhydramine, and birth control pills. There is no known drug allergy. She does not smoke cigarettes or drink alcohol.

On Physical Exam, the patient is mildly icteric but appears well. Findings include icterus of the sclera, buccal mucosa, and skin. The exam is otherwise normal.

1. Make a problem list based on the history and physical.

You decide to order blood tests. Findings include:

CBC normal
Reticulocyte count normal
Electrolytes normal
SGOT and SGPT normal
LDH normal

Alkaline phosphatase 280	(normal 30 to 110 U/L)
Direct bilirubin 2.8	(normal 0.1 to 0.3 mg/dL)
Indirect bilirubin 0.4	(normal 0.1 to 0.7 mg/dL)

2. How do the lab data help to locate this patient's jaundice on the diagnostic template? You can use the same template as in Case 3.

3. What is the likely cause of her jaundice?

Answers for Case 4

1. Problem list

Jaundice or icterus is really the only problem. "Itching" might merit a brief mention but is almost undoubtedly (at this point in the inquiry) a manifestation of the jaundice.

2. Locating the patient's jaundice on the diagnostic template

- Direct hyperbilirubinemia with normal hemoglobin, normal LDH, and increased alkaline phosphatase implies cholestasis.
- Of possible causes of cholestasis:
  - Hepatocyte damage is unlikely with normal SGOT/SGPT.
  - Congenital causes are possible given the presentation at a relatively young age.
  - Drug: Most likely. Oral contraceptives are common offenders in this regard.
  - Toxin: No history of exposure, although these can of course be occult.
  - Severe systemic illness: Contradicted by clinical presentation.
  - Primary biliary cirrhosis: Relatively unlikely based on low prevalence in this age group.
  - Pregnancy: Uncommon with oral contraceptives, but worth consideration in a young woman.
  - Mass lesion is unlikely because of low prevalence in this age group and the patient's appearance of good health.
  - Gallstones should not cause jaundice without abdominal symptoms.
  - Stricture, tumor, and sclerosing cholangitis have a low prevalence in this setting.

3. Likely cause of this patient's jaundice

Cholestasis from oral contraceptives

Tips

1. Inferring an "innocent" cause of jaundice is based on the patient's appearance of good health, her young age, and the availability of a plausible hypothesis.
2. The likelihood arguments are based on
   - Information about the patient, such as her healthy appearance
   - Information about diseases, such as their relative prevalence
   - The availability of a hypothesis that explains all features of the illness
3. How would decisions regarding diagnosis be different if features of the clinical presentation were changed?
   - *Patient has ulcerative colitis.*
     This greatly increases the possibility of sclerosing cholangitis.
   - *Patient is febrile.*
     This increases the possibility of cholecystitis or cholangitis.
   - *Patient is not taking oral contraceptives.*
     This raises the possibility of pregnancy or of such congenital syndromes as Dubin-Johnson or Rotor's.
   - *Patient looks sick.*
     This increases the possibility of biliary obstruction.

CASE 5

Bartolo Dottore

Bartolo Dottore is a 27-year-old medical student who visits you because of sore throat, sneezing, runny nose, and fever to 101°F for 3 days. This seemed like an ordinary cold until the patient noticed that the whites of his eyes had become somewhat yellow. He felt well until then and has had no previous medical problems. He takes no medicines, has no known drug allergies, and does not smoke cigarettes or drink alcohol. He has been reading up on his case and is concerned that he may have familial Mediterranean fever.

On Physical Exam, the patient appears well. Vital signs: Temp 37.8°C orally, BP $^{124}/_{84}$, HR 68, RR 12. Findings include moderate icterus of the sclera, buccal mucosa, and skin. Mild nasal congestion and pharyngeal injection without exudate are noted. The remainder of the exam is normal.

1. Make a problem list based on the history and physical.

You decide to order blood tests. Findings include:

WBC 6.6	(normal 3.4 to 11.2 K/μL)
Hgb 12.3	(normal 14 to 18 g/dL)
Reticulocyte count 8.2	(normal 0% to 1%)
Electrolytes normal	
SGOT and SGPT normal	
LDH 530	(normal 80 to 225 U/dL)
Alkaline phosphatase 85	(normal 30 to 110 U/L)

Direct bilirubin 0.2	(normal 0.1 to 0.3 mg/dL)
Indirect bilirubin 3.5	(normal 0.1 to 0.7 mg/dL)

2. How do the lab data help to locate this patient's jaundice on the diagnostic template? You can use the same template as in Case 3.

3. What is the likely cause of his jaundice?

Answers for Case 5

1. Problem list

Jaundice or icterus
Upper respiratory symptoms (lumped or split as you will)
Low-grade fever—considered as part of respiratory infection or not
Implications of being a medical student (exposure to viral infections?)

2. Locating the patient's jaundice on the diagnostic template

Indirect hyperbilirubinemia with decreased hemoglobin, increased reticulocyte count, and increased LDH implies hemolysis.

3. Likely cause of this patient's jaundice

Although there are numerous possible causes of the hemolysis, one explanation for the occurrence of acute hemolysis in the setting of an infection is G6PD deficiency.

Tips

1. If you try to extract the maximum amount of information from the clinical data, a few extra clues emerge. As a medical student, the patient has potential exposure to viral infections and to drugs. He is also prone to overwork and fatigue, which can provoke jaundice in some forms of hemolysis, as well as in Gilbert syndrome. He appears to have Italian ancestry, which implies an increased prevalence of G6PD deficiency, favism, and thalassemia trait.

2. These are best regarded as clues—potentially useful, especially if the initial analysis is inconclusive, but too weak to drive the inquiry.

CASE 6

Morbia Prendergast

Morbia Prendergast is a 29-year-old woman who sees you to have her cholesterol checked. She feels well and has not seen a doctor since the uncomplicated birth of her second child 4 years ago. She takes no medicines, has no known drug allergies, and does not smoke cigarettes or drink alcohol. The Past Medical History, Family History, and Review of Symptoms are unremarkable.

On Physical Examination, the patient appeared well. Vital signs: Temp 37.1°C tympanic, BP $^{104}/_{64}$, HR 60. The exam was normal except for scattered petechiae over the hard palate and the shins bilaterally.

Laboratory data were as follows:

Hemoglobin 13.2	(normal 12 to 16 g/dL)
WBC 7.1	(normal 3.4 to 11.2 K/μL)
Platelets 72,000	(normal 150,000 to 400,000/μL)

1. At this point, make a problem list based on the history, physical, and laboratory data.

2. Write out a diagnostic template for thrombocytopenia.

The peripheral blood smear demonstrated normal RBC and WBC without schistocytes; platelets were moderately decreased. A bone marrow biopsy found all cell lines normal.

3. **Where on the diagnostic template does Ms. Prendergast fit?**

4. **What is your working diagnosis?**

Answers for Case 6

1. Problem list

Thrombocytopenia
Petechiae should be subsumed under this.

2. Diagnostic template for *thrombocytopenia*

- I. Decreased production (*Hallmark:* Decreased megakaryocytes in marrow)
  - A. Suppression
    1. Drug
    2. Toxin
    3. Aplasia
    4. Infection
  - B. Bone marrow replacement
    1. Myelofibrosis
    2. Myelodysplastic syndrome
    3. Hematologic malignancy
    4. Bone metastases
    5. Granulomatous disease
    6. Infiltration (amyloid, hemochromatosis)
- II. Increased destruction (*Hallmark:* Normal or increased megas in marrow)
  - A. Sequestration (Splenomegaly)
  - B. Antibody mediated (*Hallmark:* No schistocytes)
    1. Immune thrombocytopenic purpura
    2. Lupus
    3. Evans' syndrome
    4. After transfusion
    5. Drug
  - C. Consumptive (*Hallmark:* Schistocytes)
    1. Disseminated intravascular coagulation
    2. Thrombotic thrombocytopenic purpura
    3. Hemolytic uremic syndrome

4. Vasculitis
5. Prosthetic cardiac valve
6. Thrombus

III. Dilution: RBC transfusion without platelet replacement

3. Locating the case on the diagnostic template

Patient has normal megakaryocytes in the marrow and therefore has increased destruction of platelets.

The absence of splenomegaly implies that sequestration is not present. The absence of schistocytes excludes consumptive coagulopathy. There has been no transfusion.

Antibody-mediated platelet destruction is therefore present.

4. Working diagnosis

Immune thrombocytopenic purpura

Of the other causes of antibody-mediated platelet destruction:

There are no other signs of lupus.

Evans' syndrome consists of immune destruction of platelets and RBCs; the latter is not present.

There is no known drug ingestion and no transfusion.

Tips

1. Note how the diagnostic template can be constructed so that major divisions into different categories can coincide with hallmark clinical features. Such simple findings as the presence or absence of schistocytes provide major discrimination value.

2. The diagnostic process is already complete at this point. Further testing with blood tests or x-rays is completely unnecessary.

CASE 7

Eleanor Sniggle

Eleanor Sniggle is a 68-year-old woman who comes to the emergency room because of fatigue and back pain. She felt well until 5 months ago, when she slipped on the ice and developed pain in the middle of her back. The pain is worse with motion and improves transiently with heat or aspirin but has not resolved. In addition, she has noted decreased energy for 1 to 2 months. There is no fever, change in sleep or appetite, or neurologic symptom.

The Past Medical History is remarkable only for mild hypertension, controlled with diet, and for a cholecystectomy 6 years ago. She takes aspirin but no other medicines and has no known drug allergies. She does not smoke and drinks 1 to 2 glasses of wine daily. Review of Systems is notable for the new development of constipation.

On Physical Exam, the patient appears somewhat pale but is in no acute distress. Vital signs: Temp 37.9°C tympanic, BP $^{138}/_{86}$, HR 104. Findings include pallor of the conjunctivae and lips, and moderate tenderness over the midthoracic spine. The remainder of the exam is normal.

1. Make a problem list based on the history and physical.

You decide to order blood tests, with results as follows:

WBC 8.2	(normal 3.4 to 11.2 K/μL)
Hgb 8.8	(normal 14 to 18 g/dL)
Electrolytes normal	

Creatinine 2.4	(normal 0.5 to 1.5 mg/dL)
Calcium 12.8	(normal 8.5 to 10.5 mg/L)
Phosphorus 3.5	(normal 2.2 to 4.2 mg/dL)
Sedimentation rate 110	(normal 5 to 20 mm/hr)

2. Make a modified problem list based on the history, physical, and laboratory data.

3. Pick two salient problems and construct diagnostic templates for them.

4. Do these intersect? Where?

5. Do other features of the illness help to locate the case within the template?

6. Any help from a "Gestalt" approach?

Answers for Case 7

1. Problem list from the history and physical

Back pain/spine tenderness
Pallor
New constipation
Fatigue
Tachycardia
History of hypertension
History of cholecystectomy

2. Problem list from history, physical, and labs

Anemia/pallor
Hypercalcemia
Renal insufficiency
Marked elevation of sedimentation rate (ESR)
Back pain/spine tenderness
New constipation
Fatigue
History of hypertension
History of cholecystectomy

3. Diagnostic templates

As the salient problems, one could pick hypercalcemia, anemia, markedly increased ESR, renal insufficiency, or back pain. Back pain is not a very fruiful place to start, however, as the causes do not give much diagnostic discrimination.

Diagnostic Template for *Hypercalcemia*

I. Increased bone resorbtion
  A. Hyperparathyroidism
  B. Related to malignancy
    1. Ectopic parathyroid hormone (PTH): Small-cell lung cancer
    2. PTH-like substance of malignancy

3. Osteoclast activating factor
    a. Multiple myeloma
    b. Squamous cell cancers: Lung, upper airways
    c. Renal cell carcinoma
4. Bone metastases

II. Increased GI absorption
  A. Increased vitamin D
  B. Granulomatous disorders: Sarcoid, tuberculosis
  C. Familial
  D. Milk alkali syndrome

III. Decreased renal excretion
  A. Drugs: Thiazides, lithium
  B. After transplant
  C. Diuretic phase of ATN

Diagnostic Template for *Anemia*

I. Decreased production
  A. Decreased substrate
    1. Iron deficiency
    2. B_{12} deficiency
    3. Folate deficiency
    4. Other deficiency (pyridoxine, etc.)
  B. Marrow dysfunction
    1. Marrow infiltration
      a. Granuloma
      b. Tumor metastases
      c. Infiltrative metabolic disease: Amyloid, etc.
    2. Hematologic malignancy
    3. Myelofibrosis, myelodysplastic syndrome
    4. Marrow suppression
      a. Toxin
      b. Hypothyroidism
      c. "Anemia of chronic disease"
      d. Renal insufficiency

II. Increased destruction
  A. Bleeding
    1. Internal

2. External
B. Hemolysis
C. Dilution
III. Sequestration

Diagnostic Template for *ESR >100 mm/hr*
I. Infection
II. Malignancy (especially myeloma)
III. Collagen-vascular disease

Diagnostic Template for *Renal Insufficiency*
I. Prerenal
A. Systemic hypovolemia
B. Local renal hypoperfusion
C. "Decreased effective renal blood flow": Edema, congestive heart failure (CHF), cirrhosis, "third spacing"
II. Renal
A. Glomerular
1. Glomerulonephritis
2. Vasculitis
B. Tubulointerstitial
1. Pyelonephritis
2. Interstitial nephritis
3. ATN
4. Multiple myeloma
5. Hypercalcemia
III. Postrenal Obstruction

4. Points of intersection

Hypercalcemia and anemia intersect at myeloma, other cancers, and granulomatous disease.

Hypercalcemia and elevated ESR intersect at infection and myeloma.

Hypercalcemia and renal insufficiency intersect at myeloma.

Anemia and elevated ESR intersect everywhere (almost).

Anemia and renal insufficiency intersect everywhere.

Elevated ESR and renal insufficiency intersect at glomerulonephritis, vasculitis, pyelonephritis, and myeloma.

5. Locating the case within the templates

While trauma alone could account for the back pain, numerous features of the illness imply a significant medical illness. These include anemia, renal insufficiency, marked ESR elevation, and the patient's ill appearance. The two ideas that keep popping up are multiple myeloma and tuberculosis.

6. Gestalt

The constellation of anemia, back pain (note atypical location), and hypercalcemia would signal multiple myeloma for most clinicians. ESR and renal insufficiency ice the cake.

Tips

1. When numerous medical problems are present, where do you begin? Promising starting places are the findings that are:
   - Most abnormal. A hemoglobin of 11.5 mg/dL is abnormal but could be due to a host of nonspecific problems. A hemoglobin of 8.8 mg/dL is very abnormal.
   - Most specific. There are relatively few causes of hypercalcemia. Pursuing this diagnosis should be relatively economical.
   - Concept of the "essence" of a case: The feature that seems at the heart of the matter.
   - New findings carry more information. If you find that the patient's creatinine was 2.4 mg/dL 5 years ago, renal insufficiency is less likely to bring you to the core of the current situation.

- Common, chronic, nonspecific complaints—such as fatigue, malaise, lassitude, body aches, back ache, and chronic constipation—are generally not good places to start. They are more promising if there is some atypical feature (atypical location, atypical age group, unusual severity, unremitting course, failure to respond to conservative therapy, etc.).

2. Of Ms. Sniggle's problems, anemia and hypercalcemia are the most specific. ESR >100 mm/hr also has a short differential diagnosis, though it is still an imprecise test. Constipation and fatigue are too nonspecific to be of much value, although their new appearance is worrisome.
3. Complex diagnostic problems are solved by breaking them down into their components, solving the component issues, and then reassembling them.

CASE 8

Omar Deng

Omar Deng is an 8-year-old boy who is brought to the Emergency Room because of fever and rash. His father says that the patient was well until 2 days ago, when he developed fever to 100°F orally, bloodshot eyes, slight cough without sputum, and loose stools. Yesterday, his cheeks became bright red for most of the day. Today spots developed over the entire body. There has been no headache, stiff neck, dyspnea, or itching.

The Past Medical History is unremarkable. He takes no medicines and has no known drug allergies. He was born in Singapore as the son of a diplomat and has lived in Perth, Australia; Khartoum, Sudan; and Göteborg, Sweden before moving to New York 3 months ago. His father has no idea what immunizations or childhood illnesses his son may have had, but birth and development are reported as normal.

On Physical Examination, the patient looked mildly ill. Vital signs: Temp 38.6°C orally, BP 100/82, HR 100, RR 16. The exam was normal except for mild conjunctival injection without discharge and for a macular-papular eruption covering the arms, legs, and trunk but not the face, scalp, genitals, palms, or soles. Mucous membranes were not involved.

1. **Make a problem list based on the history and physical.**

2. **What are the possible causes of fever and a maculopapular eruption in children? (limit to ≤10).**

3. How do details of the case distinguish among these possibilities?

4. What is your working diagnosis?

Answers for Case 8

1. Problem list

Fever
Rash
Cough
Conjunctival injection
Loose stools
Looks ill

2. Differential diagnosis

Measles
Rubella
Varicella
Smallpox
Fifth disease (erythema infectiosum)
Roseola (exanthem subitum)
Infectious mononucleosis
Other viral infections (Coxsackie, enterovirus, reovirus, arbovirus)
Rocky Mountain Spotted Fever (RMSF)
Rickettsia pox
Syphilis
Typhoid
Drug eruption

3. Homing in

Measles. Possible; however, measles usually begins on the forehead. Cough should be more prominent.

Rubella. Rubella too usually begins on the forehead. Lymphadenopathy should be present.

Varicella. Possible; however, itching should be more pronounced. Lesions in varying stages of development, including vesicles, should be seen.

Smallpox. Presumed to be eliminated, although patient's travel history might raise the question. Eruption should be vesicular, however.

Fifth Disease (Erythema Infectiosum). The best fit. The red cheeks seen on the day before the eruption is "classic" for the illness, a common infection of children in this age group. This feature makes the "cluster": a febrile exanthem preceded by mild prodrome and bright red cheeks.

Roseola. Not quite right; roseola occurs mainly in infants, and the fever disappears when the rash appears.

Infectious Mononucleosis. Imaginative, but pharyngitis and lymphadenopathy should be more prominent. A macular rash appears in 5% of cases.

Other Viral Infections. Certainly possible, but none are known for the "slapped cheek."

Rocky Mountain Spotted Fever. Imaginative, but the rash is wrong.

Rickettsia Pox. The first cases were described in New York City, so that this should not be dismissed as a third-world disease. Sparing of the palms and soles is characteristic, as in our patient. The initial papule at the site of the mite bite, a hallmark of the disease, might have been missed. However, the rash should follow a week of fever, which was not present here. The illness's low prevalence argues against it as well.

Syphilis. The patient's age does not disqualify him from secondary syphilis, but the rash is wrong; palm and sole involvement should predominate.

Scrub Typhus. Travel history is suggestive, but absence of headache and lymphadenopathy make this unlikely.

Typhoid Fever. Possible. Fever is generally higher and is accompanied by chills and headache. The hallmark is prolonged fever; perhaps we are seeing Omar early in the course. However, he has been in New York for longer than the incubation period.

Drug Eruption. The rash is right, but there is no history of drug ingestion.

4. Working diagnosis

Fifth disease

Tips

1. The diagnostic technique here involves identifying the major issues (fever and maculopapular rash), elucidating the possible causes of this combination, and then matching the diseases to the clinical presentation. Many of the diseases give an approximate fit; only Fifth disease fits well.
2. If the case read, "slapped-cheek appearance," many students would jump to the right answer immediately. They are recognizing a *verbal* constellation. The trick here is to recognize that the bright red cheeks are in fact the slapped-cheek appearance that you read about.
3. A clinician could "get by" by calling the illness a "nonspecific viral syndrome," without making a specific diagnosis. This would be therapeutically valid, in that no specific treatment is necessary here, but intellectually weak. Note that if a disease like RMSF were incorrectly tagged as a "nonspecific viral syndrome," the patient could well die.

CASE 9

*Bunter Frill**

Bunter Frill is a 68-year-old man who comes to the Urgent Care Center because of difficulty walking. He says that he felt well until 4 weeks ago, when he noticed difficulty buttoning his shirt and signing his name, "like my fingers wouldn't do what they were supposed to." Three weeks ago he developed difficulty walking, described as a tendency to stumble, especially on uneven surfaces, and his wife noticed facial grimacing. He now feels that his limbs move spontaneously, without his control; this increases after drinking coffee and decreases after drinking beer.

The Past Medical History is otherwise unremarkable. He takes no medicines and has no known drug allergies. He does not smoke and drinks 1 to 2 beers daily. He works as repose analyst at a mattress factory and is married without children. Family History is notable for Parkinson's disease in his sister, who lives with him. Review of Systems is notable for knee and ankle pain 1 month ago that lasted 1 week and resolved.

On Physical Examination, the patient appeared well. Vital signs: Temp 36.7°C orally, BP 132/82, HR 76, RR 14. Neurologic exam demonstrated brief, spontaneous, nonrhythmic, irregular, jerky movements of the face and limbs bilaterally. These occurred unpredictably and could not be initiated or stopped by the patient. They increased with fatigue or anxiety and were absent during sleep. The remainder of the physical and neurologic exam was normal.

---

*This is a true case from a prominent teaching hospital a few years ago. After much calculation and deliberation by interns, residents, attendings, and consultants, the diagnosis was suggested by a third-year medical student doing his clerkship.

1. Make a problem list based on the history and physical.
2. What is the differential diagnosis of his main problem, using a systems approach?
3. What do you think are the most likely possibilities at this point?
4. Would you recommend any tests to evaluate these possibilities?

Answers for Case 9

1. Problem list

Movement disorder
This should be identified as chorea.
History of arthralgia
(Sister with Parkinson's disease)

2. Differential Diagnosis of *chorea* (systems approach)

1. *Congenital/Genetic*	Huntington's disease Wilson's disease After birth anoxia (Paroxysmal chorea) (Hereditary acanthocytosis)
2. *Mechanical/Traumatic*	None
3. *Infectious*	Viral encephalitis
4. *Neoplastic*	None
5. *Immunologic*	Sydenham's chorea
6. *Metabolic*	Hyperthyroidism (rare) Kernicterus
7. *Vascular*	Stroke (of subthalamic nuclei)
8. *Toxic*	Drug effects: Phenothiazines, L-dopa
9. *Nutritional*	None
10. *Degenerative*	Some cases of Alzheimer's disease Some cases of Pick's disease

11. *Psychogenic*	None; choreiform movements are sometimes attributed to psychiatric disturbances in children
12. *Unknown*	Why not?

3. Most likely possibilities

Sydenham's chorea fits the bill nicely. Although no history of pharyngitis is reported, this may have been no more than a sore throat 3 to 4 months previously. The arthralgias fit the picture of rheumatic fever.

Huntington's disease should present earlier in life.

Wilson's disease should present earlier in life; Kayser-Fleischer rings are said to be always present with CNS involvement.

Viral encephalitis is an acute, febrile illness.

Hyperthyroidism should have other findings.

Stroke should have abrupt onset and gradually improve.

Drug: Has he been getting into his sister's L-dopa?

Alzheimer's or Pick's diseases: Possible, although the onset is rather too rapid for these.

4. Diagnostic tests

An antistreptolysin-O titre would confirm Sydenham's chorea.

Tips

1. The key to this case is the correct identification of the abnormal movements as chorea. To elaborate

differential diagnoses of tremor, athetosis, ataxia, seizure, myoclonus, cerebellar dysfunction, clumsiness, or other neurologic processes is to bark up the wrong tree. The involuntary movements are the "core" or "essence" of the case. Other features are subsidiary and nonspecific.

2. Even complex, unfamiliar clinical presentations yield to methodical diagnostic reasoning.

CASE 10

Rex Plover

Rex Plover is a 51-year-old man who is admitted for arthroscopic knee surgery following a tennis injury. On your admission physical examination, you detect a 2-cm plaque on the right scapula that is erythematous, scaling, irregular, and nontender. The patient has never noticed this before and feels well. The Past Medical History is notable only for the knee injury 4 months ago. The remainder of the history and physical are unremarkable.

You are trying to decide what the lesion might be and whether to recommend excisional biopsy.

You refer to the following study.[2] In the study, conducted at a university center, men and women between the ages of 40 and 65 who presented with erythematous lesions of diameters 1 to 4 cm underwent excisional biopsy. Before the biopsy, general internists at the center examined the lesions and judged whether they were benign or malignant.

There were 1200 patients enrolled in the study. The clinicians judged 150 lesions to be malignant; of these, 110 proved malignant on biopsy. A total of 130 biopsies were positive for malignancy.

1. What is the prevalence of malignancy in this study?

2. What is the sensitivity of physician examination for detecting malignancy in this study?

---

[2]Kusch, SC and Bettman, HW: Artzlichere Urteilkraft bei den dermatologischen Verletzungen. Fort. Mediz. Blödsinn 1:3–16, 1994.

3. What is the specificity of physician exam?

4. If a clinician judges a lesion to be malignant, what is the likelihood that he or she is correct?

5. You think that your patient's lesion is benign. What is the likelihood that you are correct?

6. You recommend that no biopsy be performed. Mr. Plover asks you what the probability is that he actually has skin cancer and that you missed the diagnosis.

Answers for Case 10

Begin by making a 2 × 2 Table.

Data Given in Case

N = 1200
150 lesions judged to be malignant (total positive tests)
110 of the positive tests were true positives (TP)
130 biopsies were positive for malignancy (total gold-standard positive)

	Gold Std Pos	Gold Std Neg	
Test Pos	110		150
Test Neg			
	130		1200

Calculated Data (Calculated Figures in *Italics*)

	Gold Std Pos	Gold Std Neg	
Test Pos	110	*40*	150
Test Neg	*20*	*1030*	*1050*
	130	*1070*	1200

1. Prevalence of malignancy

Prevalence = Gold Std Pos/N = (TP + FN)/N = (110 + 20)/1200 = 10.8%

2. Sensitivity of physician examination

Sensitivity = True Pos Tests/Total Gold Std Pos = TP/(TP + FN) = 110/(110 + 20) = 84.6%

3. Specificity of physcian examination

Specificity = True Neg Tests/Total Gold Std Neg = TN/(FP + TN) = 1030/(40 + 1030) = 96.3%

4. If the physician judges the lesion to be malignant, the probability that the lesion is malignant is:

Posttest probability for positive test = PTP(+) = True Pos Tests/Total Pos Tests = TP/(TP + FP) = 110/(110 + 40) = 73.3%

5. If the physician judges the lesion to be benign, the probability that the lesion is benign is:

Posttest probability of no disease with negative test = True Neg Tests/Total Neg Tests = TN/(FN + TN) = 1030/(20 + 1030) = 98.1%

6. If the physician judges the lesion to be benign, the probability that the lesion is malignant is

Posttest probability of disease with negative test = PTP(−) = FN/(FN + TN) = 20/(20 + 1030) = 1.9%

Tips

1. Let's say that you judge a lesion to be benign. What should be done? There are three possible courses:

- Reassure the patient and reevaluate in 1 year.
  This is based in the 98% probability that there is no malignancy.
- Biopsy
  This is based on the 2% chance that a malignancy is present and that you or the patient find this chance unacceptable.
- Reevaluate in 3 to 6 months.
  This splits the odds, based on the premise that a malignancy might declare itself by changing a bit and calling for biopsy then.

The best option depends on the natural history of the potential malignancy. If we were concerned about melanoma, the lesion should be excised. Melanoma can metastasize early, a fatal consequence. A 2% margin of error is unacceptable. If we were concerned about basal cell or squamous cell carcinoma, however, a "watch and wait" strategy becomes more reasonable. These malignancies should not change from minor to major in a short time period.

2. Remember that, before the physician looked at the lesion, the probability of malignancy was about 11%, the prevalence of malignancy in the study. Physician judgment "positive" changed this probability to 73%; judgment "negative," to 2%.

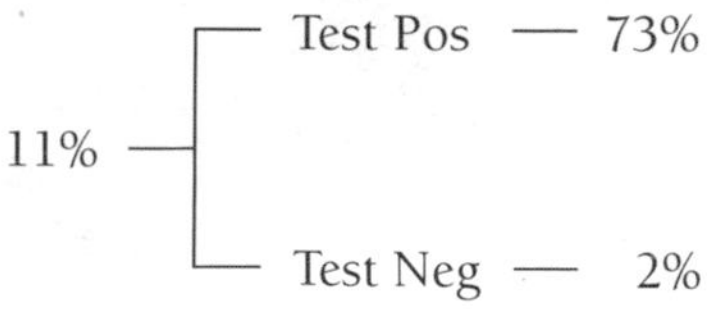

Physician judgment was a fairly discriminating test. Discriminating enough? Good enough to obviate biopsy?

3. Even good tests are quite imperfect.

CASE 11

Mamie Kriebel

Mamie Kriebel is a 62-year-old woman who consults you because her next door neighbor has been diagnosed with colon cancer. She has read about tumor markers and would like to obtain a carcinoembryonic antigen (CEA) level.

You review the literature on CEA and obtain the following information:

1. In a large study,[3] serum CEA was measured in 203 patients with known colon cancer immediately before initial surgery. CEA $\geq$2.5 ng/mL was considered positive and CEA $<$2.5 ng/mL was considered negative. By this standard, 91 patients with cancer had positive CEA and 112 had negative CEA.
2. The prevalence of colon cancer in asymptomatic, 60-year-old Americans is approximately 1 per 1000.[4]
3. The specificity of CEA testing for Dukes A or B cancer is approximately 87%.[5]

1. What is the sensitivity of CEA for patients of this sort?

---

[3]Wanebo, HI, et al: Preoperative carcinoembryonic antigen level as a prognostic indicator in colorectal cancer. N Engl J Med 299: 448–451, 1978.

[4]Greegor, DH: Detection of silent colon cancer in routine examination. CA Cancer J Clin 19:330–337, 1969.

[5]Liu, YS, et al: A more specific, simpler radioimmunoassay for carcinoembryonic antigen, with use of monoclonal antibodies. Clin Chem 31:191–195, 1985.

2. If Ms. Kriebel's CEA is positive, what is the probability that she has colon cancer?

3. If her CEA is negative, what is the probability that she has colon cancer anyway?

4. Would you recommend a CEA test? Why or why not?

5. Ms. Kriebel now tells you that three of her four siblings developed colon cancer. This may increase the risk of colon cancer tenfold. Would you now recommend CEA testing? There is no history of familial polyposis or inflammatory bowel disease

6. Why is the specificity for Dukes A and B cancer given, instead of all stages?

Answers for Case 11

For this 2 × 2 table, the population of interest is a hypothetical group of middle-aged Americans at average risk of colon cancer. The CEA study involves 203 patients who are all gold-standard positive.

Data Given in Study

	Gold Std Pos	Gold Std Neg
Test Pos	91	
Test Neg	112	
	203	

To complete the table:

1. Calculate the total population N. If 203 persons have cancer, and 1 person in 1000 has cancer, the total population we are considering has N = 203 × 1000 = 203,000.
2. Total without cancer = 203,000 − 203 = 202,797.
3. Calculate True Negatives (TN) using specificity. TN = spec × total without cancer = 0.87 × 202,797 = 176,433.
4. Complete the table by additions and subtractions.

Calculated Data (Calculated Figures in *Italics*)

	Gold Std Pos	Gold Std Neg	
Test Pos	91	*26,364*	*26,455*
Test Neg	112	*176,433*	*176,545*
	203	*202,797*	*203,000*

1. Sensitivity of CEA for this population

Sensitivity = 91/203 = 44.8%

2. Probability of cancer with positive CEA

Posttest probability of disease with positive test = PPT(+) = 91/26,455 = 0.3%

3. Probability of cancer with negative CEA

Posttest probability of disease with negative test = PTP(−) = 112/176,545 = 0.06%

4. Recommend CEA?

No. Less than 1% of asymptomatic persons with positive tests will actually have cancer. Put another way, almost all the positive tests are false positives. It *is* true that a negative test implies a very low probability of cancer; but it only reduces the probability from 0.10% to 0.06%!

5. 2 × 2 table for prevalence of 1%

	Gold Std Pos	Gold Std Neg	
Test Pos	91	2,613	2,704
Test Neg	112	17,484	17,596
	203	20,097	20,300

Probability of cancer with positive CEA = PTP(+)
= 91/2704 = 3.4%

Probability of cancer with negative CEA = PTP(−)
= 112/17,596 = 0.6%

As the prevalence increases, the significance of a positive test increases too. However, even for this high prevalence group, the significance of a positive test has increased only slightly. The majority of persons with positive tests will not have colon cancer. The test is still not recommended.

6. Why are we talking about Dukes A and B cancers only?

A screening test is valuable only if it detects disease at a time when intervention changes the course of the disease favorably. Early detection of Dukes C or D cancer is not beneficial to the patient.

Tips

1. CEA is not an effective screening test. Since a person with no special risk for colon cancer has a pretest probability of 0.1% for having the disease, a positive CEA increases the probability to only

0.3%. A negative CEA decreases the probability to only 0.06%.

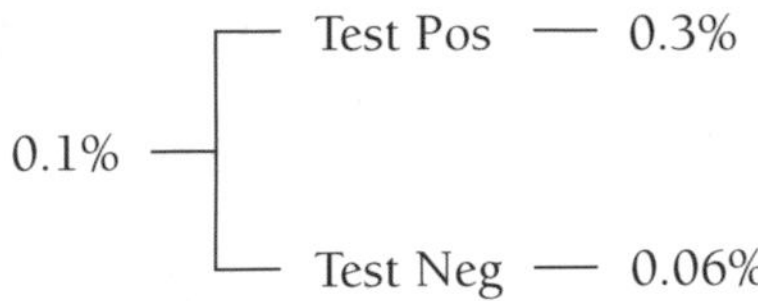

Performing the test has taught us very little about the patient.

2. Since a negative test implies a very low probability of cancer, couldn't CEA be used to reassure people? If you think yes, how would you feel if you were one of the people with a positive CEA who then had to undergo a (negative) search for cancer, which would include colonoscopy and perhaps more?
3. A screening test should lead to as few false positives as possible. When CEA is used as a screening test, almost all the positive tests are false positives. This does not negate the role of CEA in following certain patients with known adenocarcinoma. But CEA should not be used for screening.

CASE 12

Hans Castorp

Hans Castorp is a 48-year-old man who comes to the Emergency Department because of fever and cough for 5 weeks. He reports no previous medical problems, takes no medicines, has no known drug allergies. He smokes cigars, drinks socially, and reports no HIV risk factors. He worked as an investment banker but retired at age 41, divorced at age 42, and has no children. Review of Systems is notable for a 10-lb weight loss over the last month.

On Physical Exam, he appears somewhat ill and is coughing. Vital signs: Temp 38.8°C orally, BP 130/88, HR 100, RR 22. Findings include poor dentition, 1-cm axillary lymphadenopathy, coarse breath sounds in the right upper field, and chronic venous stasis changes over the shins bilaterally.

You are considering the diagnosis of pulmonary tuberculosis. You ask your resident about the value of performing an acid-fast bacillus (AFB) smear of the sputum and find that, while she wants you to do one, she has no idea how accurate it is. You therefore run to the library, run a quick literature search, and find the following study.[6] In the study, 1828 patients were suspected of having pulmonary tuberculosis (TB) and had sputum analyzed by both acid-fast smear and mycobacterial culture. There were 52 positive smears, of which 46 were positive by culture. In addition, 13 positive cultures had negative smears.

---

[6]Strumpf, IJ, et al: Re-evaluation of sputum staining for the diagnosis of pulmonary tuberculosis. Am Rev Resp Dis 119:599–602, 1979.

1. What is the sensitivity, in this study, of AFB smear for detecting pulmonary TB?

2. What is the specificity?

3. You estimate that, based on the clinical picture alone, the probability of pulmonary TB is about 25%. If the smear is positive, what is the probability that Mr. Castorp has pulmonary TB? If the smear is negative, what is the probability that he still has TB?

As you try to collect a sputum sample, Mr. Castorp confides to you that he lost his job because of alcoholism and that he has been living on the streets for almost a year.

4. Based on this new information, you increase your estimate of the clinical probability of TB to 80%. If the smear is positive, what is the probability of TB? If the smear is negative, what is the probability of TB?

5. The smear is negative. The ER attending wants to discharge the patient and arrange for outpatient follow-up in the Pulmonary Clinic. What do you think?

Answers for Case 12

Data Given in Case

N = 1828
52 positive smears (total positive tests); 46 of these had positive cultures (true positives)
13 negative smears had positive cultures (false negatives)

	Gold Std Pos	Gold Std Neg	
Test Pos	46		52
Test Neg	13		
			1828

Calculated Data (Calculated Figures in *Italics*)

	Gold Std Pos	Gold Std Neg	
Test Pos	46	6	52
Test Neg	13	*1763*	*1776*
	59	*1769*	1828

1. Sensitivity of smear for TB

Sensitivity = 46/59 = 78.0%

2. Specificity of smear for TB

$$\text{Specificity} = 1763/1769 = \underline{99.7\%}$$

Now we know about the *test*, AFB smear—that is, we know how the AFB smear compares with a gold standard. We still don't know anything about the *patient*.

3. Probability of TB with positive or negative smear

Step 1

To calculate posttest probability, assume a hypothetical sample of 1000 patients resembling the index patient. If the pretest probability of disease is 25%, there are 250 patients who are gold-standard positive.

	Gold Std Pos	Gold Std Neg	
Test Pos			
Test Neg			
	250	750	1000

Step 2

Of the 250 patients who are gold-standard positive, the number who test positive is 250 × sensitivity = 195.

Similarly, of the 750 patients who are gold-standard negative, the number who test negative is 750 × specificity = 748.

	Gold Std Pos	Gold Std Neg	
Test Pos	*195*		
Test Neg		*748*	
	250	750	1000

Step 3

With a little more arithmetic:

	Gold Std Pos	Gold Std Neg	
Test Pos	*195*	*2*	*197*
Test Neg	*55*	*748*	*803*
	250	750	1000

Probability of TB with positive test = PTP(1)

= 195/197 = 98.9%

Probability of TB with negative test = PTP(2)

= 55/803 = 6.8%

4. Probability of TB with pretest probability 80% and with positive or negative smear

With a pretest probability of 80%:

	Gold Std Pos	Gold Std Neg	
Test Pos	*624*	*1*	*625*
Test Neg	*176*	*199*	*375*
	800	200	1000

Probability of TB with positive test = PTP(+)
= 624/625 = <u>99.8%</u>

Probability of TB with negative test = PTP(−)
= 176/375 = <u>46.9%</u>

5. Management decision for patient with pretest probability 80% but negative smear

With a negative smear, the patient still has a 47% probability of TB. A homeless man with this chance of TB cannot be discharged.

Tips

1. Observe how the estimation of pretest probability affects the interpretation of the test. When the pretest probability was 25%, a negative test conferred a posttest probability of 7%. When the pretest probability was 80%, a negative test conferred a posttest probability of 47%.
2. Note that the PPD is a good test. A pretest probability of 25% goes to 99% if the test is positive or to 7% if the test is negative. The test changes the pretest probability a lot.
3. Are our gold standards always the best points of

reference? If a patient has a positive smear but a negative culture, does that mean that the smear was wrong? Perhaps the culture was wrong—as could happen if the specimen were handled poorly, or if culture conditions were imperfect. One wonders whether a different gold standard, such as polymerase chain reaction, would be more reliable—in which case the AFB smear would have fewer false positives and the specificity would increase.

4. Your role as a student or house officer is not to execute someone else's directives but to think for yourself. You have a unique vantage on a clinical case and will often be unencumbered by habit, enabling you to reason through the situation.

CASE 13

Ludmilla T. Raum

Ludmilla T. Raum is a 36-year-old woman who consults you because of fever, cough, and malaise for 6 weeks. There has been low-grade fever but no sputum, chest pain, or dyspnea. The Past Medical History is unremarkable. She takes no medicines, has no known drug allergies, smokes 1 ppd, and does not drink alcohol. There is no known HIV risk factor.

On Physical Examination, the patient appears well. Vital Signs: Temperature 38.1°C orally, BP 110/74, HR 88, RR 18. The exam is normal except for a palpable spleen tip. CBC and profile are normal. Chest x-ray reveals bilateral hilar adenopathy and increased interstitial markings in the perihilar region.

You are considering the possibility of sarcoidosis and collect the following figures for three diagnostic tests, based on their ability to detect stage 2 sarcoid.

Test	Sensitivity	Specificity
Transbronchial biopsy (TBB)	80%	99%
Open lung biopsy (OLB)	97%	99%
Angiotensin converting enzyme (ACE)	77%	50%

1. If the pretest probability of sarcoidosis is 50%, what is the posttest probability for each of the tests if the test is positive? What if the test is negative?

2. The ACE level is a blood test with minimal morbidity. TBB is a bronchoscopic procedure with mild-to-moderate morbidity. OLB is a surgical procedure with moderate morbidity. Which test would you choose for your patient?

3. You discover that Ms. Raum used IV drugs in the late 1980s and has lost 15 lb. Reasoning that she may have HIV infection with *Pneumocystis* pneumonia, you reduce the pretest probability of sarcoid to 20%. The ACE level is positive. What is the probability of sarcoid?

Answers for Case 13

1. Probability of disease for positive and negative results in each test

Transbronchial Biopsy

CALCULATED DATA (CALCULATED FIGURES IN *ITALICS*)

	Gold Std Pos	Gold Std Neg	
Test Pos	*400*	5	*405*
Test Neg	*100*	*495*	*595*
	500	500	1000

PTP(+) = 400/45 = <u>98.8%</u>

PTP(−) = 100/595 = <u>16.8%</u>

Open Lung Biopsy

CALCULATED DATA (CALCULATED FIGURES IN *ITALICS*)

	Gold Std Pos	Gold Std Neg	
Test Pos	*485*	5	*490*
Test Neg	*15*	*495*	*510*
	500	500	1000

$$PTP(+) = 485/490 = \underline{99.0\%}$$

$$PTP(-) = 15/510 = \underline{2.9\%}$$

Angiotensin Converting Enzyme Level

CALCULATED DATA (CALCULATED FIGURES IN *ITALICS*)

	Gold Std Pos	Gold Std Neg	
Test Pos	*385*	*250*	*635*
Test Neg	*115*	*250*	*365*
	500	500	1000

$$PTP(+) = 385/635 = \underline{60.6\%}$$

$$PTP(-) = 115/365 = \underline{31.5\%}$$

2. Which test?

TBB provides less information than OLB, but it has considerably less morbidity. A positive TBB would confirm the diagnosis, while a negative test leaves a modest possibility of missed sarcoid.

OLB does no better than TBB on PTP(+) but has a significantly lower false-negative rate. This is purchased at the cost of increased morbidity.

ACE level only changes the pretest probability from 50% to 61% if positive or to 31% if negative. A test is most useful when its result changes the pretest probability the most. If a test, such as the ACE level, doesn't affect probabilities much whether positive or negative, don't order the test.

3. For pretest probability of 20%, the 2 × 2 table for ACE is as follows:

	Gold Std Pos	Gold Std Neg	
Test Pos	*154*	*400*	*554*
Test Neg	*46*	*400*	*446*
	200	800	1000

PTP(+) = 154/554 = 27.8%

The ACE level has changed the probability of sarcoid hardly at all.

Tips

1. Test results like the positive ACE level in question 3 occur all the time, going by such names as "red herring" and "false lead" and "lab error." Don't be misled by positive tests: if the pretest probability is low, or the test's specificity is low, the posttest probability may be low even with a positive test. Doctors who are not clear on this concept often feel obliged to perform further testing in order to "rule out" sarcoid.
2. The best test is the one that gives the greatest splay in probabilities between positive and negative results, for the least morbidity and cost. TBB fits the bill here. One must be mindful, however, that demanding less morbidity may mean accepting less sensitivity. TBB is more likely than OLB to yield a false negative. For a pretest probability of 25%, a

negative TBB still confers a 17% chance of sarcoid, while a negative OLB confers a 2% chance of sarcoid.

At this stage of the evaluation, TBB is the preferred test. But if the test is negative, and the clinical picture continues to point to sarcoid, remind yourself that you have not "ruled out" sarcoid. OLB may be necessary anyway.

CASE 14

Susan Domonas

Susan Domonas is a 31-year-old woman with systemic lupus who comes to the ambulatory medical practice because of fever and headache for 1 day. Her lupus had been fairly active for 2 weeks, with pain and swelling of her wrists and metacarpal-phalangeal (MCP) joints as well as fever to 100°. She developed runny nose and dry cough 3 days ago but had no other symptoms until today, when she awoke with severe, nonpulsatile, global headache and fever to 102°. On questioning, she does report stiff neck as well as increased pain and swelling of her joints, now involving her knees and ankles as well.

The Past Medical History is notable for lupus for 12 years, characterized by inflammatory arthritis of most large joints, malar rash, mild anemia, moderate proteinuria, and occasional pleuritic chest pain. She was last treated with glucocorticoids 2 years ago. She now takes ibuprofen 800 mg every 6 to 8 hours and has no known drug allergies. She neither smokes cigarettes nor drinks alcohol. She works as a lawyer and is unmarried. Review of Systems is notable for an 8-lb weight loss over the past 3 weeks.

On Physical Examination, the patient appeared acutely ill. Vital Signs: Temp 39.4°C rectally, BP 132/88, HR 108. Notable findings included normal optic fundi, moderate nuchal rigidity, and inflammatory changes of the MCP joints, wrists, knees, and ankles. She appeared slightly somnolent. Brudzinski's sign (hip flexion following passive neck flexion) was positive, but there were no other abnormal neurologic findings.

1. At this point, make a problem list based on the history and physical exam.

2. What are the possible causes of her main acute problem?

3. Of the following management options, which do you think is best? Why?
   a. Check blood tests and prescribe a broad-spectrum oral antibiotic.
   b. Check blood tests and administer a broad-spectrum intravenous antibiotic.
   c. Perform lumbar puncture and insist that she telephone for results the next day.
   d. Send her to the hospital Admissions Office for routine admission.
   e. Refer her to the hospital Emergency Department; recommend lumbar puncture followed immediately by IV antibiotics before any results are available.
   f. Refer her to the hospital Emergency Department; recommend lumbar puncture and wait for results before making further decisions.

Answers for Case 14

1. Problem list

Meningismus: Stiff neck, nuchal rigidity, Brudzinski's sign
Fever
Weight loss
Lupus
Upper respiratory symptoms
Ibuprofen use

2. The main acute problem is clearly the meningeal signs with fever.

The differential diagnosis includes:
- Septic meningitis
- Aseptic meningitis
- Lupus involving the CNS
- Various less likely possibilities: CNS bleed (with coincidental fever), viral syndrome (without meningeal involvement)

3. Management choices

The best choice is **e**. The patient should be taken to the Emergency Department for immediate lumbar puncture followed by immediate intravenous antibiotics.

Choices **a**, **b**, **c**, and **d** all underestimate the potential severity of her illness. If bacterial meningitis proves to be present, delay in treatment is disastrous.

Choice **f** also misses the urgency of treating possible bacterial meningitis immediately.

Tips

1. The clinician must often act before a definitive diagnosis is possible. Here, the working diagnosis is

bacterial meningitis. Every effort is made to do as much as possible for this potentially life-threatening disease. Waiting even a short time to obtain more diagnostic information is not warranted. Ordinarily, there is time to perform lumbar puncture before administering antibiotics, which are given practically as soon as the needle is removed from the back.

2. An underlying issue here is the risk-to-benefit ratio. The risk of not treating bacterial meningitis promptly exceeds the benefit of obtaining more diagnostic information.
3. For this patient, the CSF showed the following:

WBC 50	(normal 0 to 1/mL)
RBC 1	(normal 0 to 5/mL)
Protein 80	(normal 20 to 40 mg/dL)
Glucose 30	(normal 40 to 70 mg/dL)
Gram's stain	No organisms seen

Smears for AFB, fungus, and cryptococcus all negative

She was treated with broad-spectrum intravenous antibiotics and admitted to the hospital. However, her fevers, headache, and stiff neck persisted, and her joints became markedly more inflamed. The blood WBC was 14,000 without left shift, and no schistocytes were seen. Complement levels were markedly decreased. CT scan of the head was normal. Proteinuria increased to nephrotic range. Cultures of the CSF, blood, urine, and sputum remained negative. The HIV titre and PPD were negative.

On the fifth hospital day, repeat lumbar puncture showed identical findings. This result after therapy argued against bacterial meningitis, and aseptic meningitis was reconsidered. The leading diagnosis became CNS lupus. Of note, ibuprofen can also cause aseptic meningitis.

Should IV Antibiotics Be Discontinued Now? What Are the Advantages and Disadvantages of Doing So?

Advantages:	No evidence of bacterial infection at this point
	Decrease risk of side effects
Disadvantages:	Remaining uncertainty regarding the possibility of infection

Antibiotics were in fact stopped, and intravenous glucocorticoids were administered. The patient recovered rapidly.

In Retrospect, Would You Have Treated This Patient Any Differently?

Probably not. Even though she proved to have aseptic meningitis from lupus, the benefit of treating bacterial meningitis was so high, and the risk of antibiotics so relatively low, that immediate treatment was warranted.

Put another way, at the time the decision needed to be made, the possibility of bacterial meningitis was fairly high, and the risk of not treating bacterial meningitis is tremendous.

4. Ibuprofen belongs on the problem list because it can (rarely) cause aseptic meningitis.
5. When the course does not follow expectations, the clinician goes back to the differential diagnosis to reconsider options that had previously seemed unlikely.

APPENDIX A

Medical Abbreviations

General Principles

1. Abbreviations are an indispensable part of clinical life. While many are used commonly and are therefore familiar, others are used infrequently and are potentially obscure.
2. Abbreviations are best used in written language, not in speech. They should, in general, not be used in communication with patients.
3. If you are uncertain whether someone will recognize an abbreviation, don't use it. Some terms are part of a subspecialty lingo that is unfamiliar to other physicians. For example, "BRBPR" is familiar to a gastroenterologist as "bright red blood per rectum;" out of context, the term is unrecognizable.
4. Abbreviations listed here that are marked with an asterisk (*) are somewhat obscure and should be avoided.
5. Capitalization, in clinical practice, is inconsistent.

Orders and Prescriptions

Abbreviation	Meaning	Rationale
QD, qd, qD	each day, daily	*quaque die*
q 6 hr, q6h, q6hr	every 6 hours	by analogy with above

Abbreviation	Meaning	Rationale
BID	2 times a day	*bis in die*
TID	3 times a day	*ter in die*
QID, qid	4 times a day	*quater in die*
QOD	every other day	by analogy with above
QHS, qhs	at bedtime	*quaque hora somni*
*BIW (TIW)	twice weekly (thrice)	a made-up concoction
PO	orally, by mouth	*per os*
sl, SL	under the tongue, sublingually	*sub lingua*
PR	rectally	*per rectum*
IV	intravenously	
IVSS	IV slowly	IV Soluset® (a trade name)
SC, SQ	subcutaneously	
ID	intradermal	
IM	intramuscularly	
*IT	intrathecal	
PRN, prn	as needed, as circumstances require	*pro re nata*
$\bar{c}$	with	*cum*
$\bar{s}$	without	*sine*
p	after	*post*
a	before	*ante*
ac	before meals	*ante cibos*
NPO	nothing by mouth	
DAW	dispense as written	
NR	no refill	

Symptoms

Abbreviation	Meaning
CP	chest pain
HA	headache
N/V	nausea and vomiting
SOB	shortness of breath
SSCP	substernal chest pain
Sx	symptom
Sz	seizure

Physical Findings

Abbreviation	Meaning
C/C/E	cyanosis, clubbing, edema
CN	cranial nerves
DTR	deep tendon reflexes
HIF	higher intellectual function
HSM	hepatosplenomegaly
JVD, JVP	jugular venous distention, pressure
NABS	normal abdominal bowel sounds
NT	nontender
O×3	oriented × 3
PERRL(A)	pupils equal, round, reactive to light (and accommodation)
PMI	point of maximal impulse
RRR	regular rate and rhythm

Laboratory Tests

Abbreviation	Meaning
ABG	arterial blood gas
alb	albumin

Abbreviation	Meaning
alk phos	alkaline phosphatase
ALT	alanine aminotransferase
ANA	antinuclear antibody
AST	aspartate aminotransferase
bili	bilirubin
BUN	blood urea nitrogen
C3 (C4)	third complement component (4th)
CBC	complete blood count
CEA	carcinoembryonic antigen
Chol	cholesterol
CPK or CK	creatine (phospho)kinase
Cr	creatinine
ds-DNA	double-stranded DNA
Echo	echocardiogram
EKG, ECG	electrocardiogram
ESR	erythrocyte sedimentation rate
ETT	exercise tolerance test
Fe/TIBC	iron/total iron binding capacity
GGT	γ-glutamyltransferase
glu	glucose
Hct	hematocrit
Hgb	hemoglobin
indirect bili	indirect bilirubin
LDH	lactate dehydrogenase
lytes	electrolytes
MCV	mean corpuscular volume
plt	platelets
pro	protein
PSA	prostate specific antigen
RBC	red blood cell count
RF	rheumatoid factor
RNCA	radionucleotide cineangiogram
SGOT	serum glutamic-oxaloacetic transaminase
SGPT	serum glutamic-pyruvic transaminase
UA	urinalysis
WBC	white blood cell count

Radiology

Abbreviation	Meaning
AP	anterior-posterior
AXR	abdominal x-ray
BE or BaE	barium enema
CT	computed tomography
CXR	chest x-ray
IVP	intravenous pyelogram
KUB	kidney-ureter-bladder (x-ray highlighting these areas)
MRI	magnetic resonance image
PA	posterior-anterior
SBFT	small bowel follow-through
UGI	upper gastrointestinal series

Procedures and Operations

Abbreviation	Meaning
AKA (BKA)	above-the-knee amputation (below-the-knee)
AVR	aortic valve replacement
BSO	bilateral salpingo-oophorectomy
CABG	coronary artery bypass graft
cath	cardiac catheterization
cysto	cystoscopy
D & C	dilation and curettage
D & E	dilation and evacuation
ECT	electroconvulsive therapy
EGD	esophageal gastroduodenoscopy
ERCP	endoscopic retrograde cholangiopancreatography
MVR	mitral valve replacement
PTCA	percutaneous transluminal coronary angioplasty
SAB	spontaneous abortion

Abbreviation	Meaning
TAB	therapeutic abortion
TAH	total abdominal hysterectomy
*TKR	total knee replacement
*THR	total hip replacement
TURB	transurethral resection of the bladder
TURP	transurethral resection of the prostate

Diagnoses

Abbreviation	Meaning
AIN	acute interstitial nephritis
ALL	acute lymphocytic leukemia
AML	acute myelogenous leukemia
ARDS	adult respiratory distress syndrome
ARF	acute renal failure
ATN	acute tubular necrosis
*CFS	chronic fatigue syndrome
CHF	congestive heart failure
CLL	chronic lymphocytic leukemia
CML	chronic myelogenous leukemia
COPD	chronic obstructive pulmonary disease
*CRI	chronic renal insufficiency
CVA	cerebrovascular accident
DIC	disseminated intravascular coagulation
DVT	deep vein thrombosis
Dx	diagnosis
*GERD	gastroesophageal reflux disease
IBD	inflammatory bowel disease
MI	myocardial infarction
PE	pulmonary embolism
PID	pelvic inflammatory disease
PUD	peptid ulcer disease
SAH	subarachnoid hemorrhage
SDH	subdural hematoma

Medications

Abbreviation	Meaning
*APAP	acetaminophen
ASA	aspirin
AZT	zidovudine
*CEI	converting enzyme inhibitor (ACE inhibitor)
DDAVP	arginine vasopressin (l-desamino-8-D-arginine vasopressin)
DDC	dideoxycytosine
DDI	dideoxyinosine
DHPG	ganciclovir
*DOCC	docusate sodium
Epo	erythropoietin
FFP	fresh frozen plasma
G-CSF	granulocyte colony stimulating factor
INH	isoniazid
MOM	milk of magnesia
MSO_4	morphine sulfate
NTG	nitroglycerin
NTP	nitropaste (nitroglycerin ointment)
*PCA	procainamide
PCN	penicillin
PRBC	packed red blood cells (blood transfusion)
PZA	pyrazinamide
*QSO_4	quinidine sulfate
TCA	tricyclic antidepressant
*TCN	tetracycline
TMP-SMX	trimethoprim-sulfamethoxazole
TPA	tissue plasminogen activator

APPENDIX B

Readings and References

Manuals

Ferri, FF: Practical Guide to the Care of the Medical Patient, ed 2. CV Mosby, St Louis, 1991. A good pocket manual, including work-up, differential diagnosis, and management of common inpatient problems.

Woodley, M and Whelan, A: Manual of Medical Therapeutics (Washington Manual), ed 27. Little, Brown & Co, Boston, 1992. The intern's standard guide to patient management.

Haist, SA, Robbins, JB, and Gomella, LG: Internal Medicine on Call, ed 2. Appleton & Lange, Norwalk, CT, 1993. A problem-based guide to patient management, emphasizing immediate care of inpatient situations. Includes good section on laboratory tests.

Macklin, RM, Mendelsohn, ME, and Mudge, Jr, GH: Manual of Introductory Clinical Medicine, ed 3. Little, Brown & Co, Boston, 1994. A synopsis of history taking, physical examination, laboratory tests, and *very* basic pathophysiology.

Textbooks of Medicine

Cecil's and Harrison's remain the standard medical textbooks. The *Scientific American* text is also excellent, providing frequent updates, and is available on-line. All three publish condensed versions; these follow the outlines of the complete versions and can therefore lead readily into the full texts.

Harvey, AM, et al: The Principles and Practice of Medicine, ed 22. Appleton & Lange, Norwalk, CT, 1988. A good student text, emphasizing clinical presentations somewhat more than diseases.

Fishman, MC, et al: Medicine, ed 3. JB Lippincott, Philadelphia, 1991. Brevity is achieved by sketchy descriptions rather than concision. Popular among third-year students, but unlikely to prove useful afterward.

Differential Diagnosis and Diagnosis

Samiy, AH, Douglas, Jr, RG, and Barondess, JA: Textbook of Diagnostic Medicine. Lea & Febiger, Philadelphia, 1987. The best text and reference for differential diagnosis.

Barondess, JA and Carpenter, CCJ: Differential Diagnosis. Lea & Febiger, Philadelphia, 1994. This new volume is organized according to clinical problem and includes discussion of each of the diagnostic possibilities. Cases chosen from the *New England Journal of Medicine*, clinico-pathologic conferences are used as illustrations and demonstrations.

Barrows, HS and Pickell, GC: Developing Clinical Problem-Solving Skills: A Guide to More Effective Diagnosis and Treatment. WW Norton, New York, 1991. An analysis and how-to of clinical problem solving, from a major leader in medical education.

Kassirer, JP and Kopelman, RI: Learning Clinical Reasoning. Williams & Wilkins, Baltimore, 1991. Another excellent approach to the diagnostic process and decision making, from the editor of *The New England Journal of Medicine.* The heart of the book consists of case analysis, how the thinking proceeded and how it went right or wrong.

Friedman, HH: Problem-Oriented Medical Diagnosis, ed 5. Little, Brown & Co, Boston, 1991. A good manual for differential diagnosis.

Adler, SN et al: A Pocket Manual of Differential Diagnosis, ed 3. Little, Brown & Co., Boston, 1994. A list approach to differential diagnosis.

Walker, HK, Hall, WD, and Hurst, JW: Clinical Methods: The History, Physical, and Laboratory Examinations, ed 3. Butterworths, Boston, 1990. An excellent reference for all aspects of diagnosis.

Cutler, P: Problem Solving in Clinical Medicine, ed 2. Williams & Wilkins, Baltimore, 1985. A good overview of clinical process using traditional methods.

Johns, RJ and Fortuin, NG: The analysis and synthesis of clinical information. In Harvey AM, et al (eds): The Principles and Practice of Medicine, ed 22. Appleton & Lange, Norwalk, CT, 1988, pp 22–24. A nice three-page overview of clinical process.

Fulop, M: Teaching differential diagnosis to beginning clinical students. Am J Med 79:745, 1985. A good presentation of the "Systems" approach to differential diagnosis.

Aronson, MD and Delbanco, TL: Manual of Clinical Evaluation: Strategies for Cost-Effective Care. Little, Brown & Co, Boston, 1988. A condensed outline of differential diagnosis and management for common disorders. More attention to sensitivity, specificity, and cost than most other books. Some of the clinical recommendations are idiosyncratic, however.

Cope, Z: The Early Diagnosis of the Acute Abdomen, ed 6. Oxford University Press, London, 1932. A classic treatise of differential diagnosis, important not only for its analysis of a common clinical presentation but for its approach to the diagnostic process.

Diagnostic Testing

Sox, HC: Common Diagnostic Tests: Use and Interpretation, ed 2. American College of Physicians, Philadelphia, 1990. Rational use of common diagnostic tests. The emphasis is on the demonstration of efficacy rather than simple conventional usage.

Panzer, R et al: Diagnostic Strategies for Common Medical Problems. American College of Physicians, Philadelphia, 1991. An excellent reference for working up cases rationally. Uses representative clinical problems and does not try to be exhaustive.

Wallace, J: Interpretation of Diagnostic Tests: A Synopsis of Laboratory Medicine, ed 5. Little, Brown & Co, Boston, 1992. An outline of test values and what they mean; somewhat ungainly.

Sacher, RA and McPherson, RA: Widmann's Clinical Interpretation of Laboratory Tests, ed 10. FA Davis, Philadelphia, 1991. A comprehensive account of blood and urine tests, including both the interpretation of tests and the physiology underlying them.

Fischbach, F: A Manual of Diagnostic Tests, ed 4. JB Lippincott, Philadelphia, 1992. Well chosen, valuable information. Organized by the test; not well cross-indexed by disease or problem.

Henry, JB: Clinical Diagnosis and Management by Laboratory Methods, ed 18. WB Saunders, Philadelphia, 1991. A reference for laboratory tests—How they are performed, confounding factors, etc.

Using the Medical Literature

Fletcher, RH, Fletcher, SW, and Wagner, EH: Clinical Epidemiology: The Essentials, ed 2. Williams & Wilkins, Baltimore, 1988. An excellent, concise description of the material.

Sackett, DL et al: Clinical Epidemiology: A Basic Science for Clinical Medicine, ed 2. Little, Brown & Co, Boston, 1991. An excellent analysis and guide for rational patient management.

Gehlbach, SH: Interpreting the Medical Literature, ed 3. McGraw-Hill, New York, 1993. A good, purposeful synopsis.

Electrocardiography

Wagner, GS: Marriott's Practical Electrocardiography, ed 9. Williams & Wilkins, Baltimore, 1994. The most reliable EKG text. The author has collaborated with Henry Marriott, who wrote the first eight editions of the text, in producing this updated and revised version.

Scheidt, S, with contributions by Erlebacher, JA: Basic Electrocardiography. CIBA, West Caldwell, NJ, 1986. An excellent and concise guide, illustrated by the famous Frank H. Netter.

Dubin, D: Rapid Interpretation of EKGs, ed 4. Cover Publishing Co, Tampa, 1989. A popular beginner's guide. Good to read once, but simplified more than necessary, and therefore not useful in future years.

Davis, D: How to Quickly and Accurately Master ECG Interpretation. JB Lippincott, Philadelphia, 1985. Very basic, but the tracings are exceptionally clear. Split infinitives in the title, and the like, might make some readers cringe.

Thaler, MS: The Only EKG Book You'll Ever Need. JB Lippincott, Philadelphia, 1988. Good. More cardiology than the other handbooks and more likely to be useful in future years.

Procedures

Vander Salm, TJ, et al (eds): Atlas of Bedside Procedures, ed 2. Little, Brown & Co., Boston, 1988. Clear descriptions and drawings of how to do the common procedures.

Gerberding, JL: Protecting healthcare workers from HIV infection. Contemporary Internal Medicine. February, 1991, p 45.

Drugs and Therapy

American Hospital Formulary Service Drug Information. Annual editions. American Society of Hospital Pharmacists, Bethesda, MD, 1995. A compendium of objective, unbiased information on essentially all drugs.

Drug Facts and Comparisons. Annual editions. Facts & Comparisons, St Louis, 1995. Another excellent reference, comprehensive and impartial. It is revised and published annually.

Physician's Desk Reference (PDR). Annual editions. Medical Economics Data Production Company, Montvale, NJ, 1995. An annual compilation of *what pharmaceutical companies say about their products*. It is not as clear as *American Hospital Formulary* or *Drug Facts and Comparisons* on such topics as mechanisms of action, side effects, and comparison with other agents. Separate *PDR*s are published for over-the-counter medications, ophthalmic preparations, and drug side effects and interactions.

The Medical Letter on Drugs and Therapeutics. Drugs of Choice. The Medical Letter, Inc., New Rochelle,

NY, 1993. A concise, impartial guide to common classes of medications. Not all classes of medication are covered.

Sanford, JP: Guide to Antimicrobial Therapy 1995. Antimicrobial Therapy, Dallas, 1995. An annually published pocket handbook for management of infectious diseases. The one item, besides a stethoscope, that most residents on medicine or surgery keep in their pockets. A similar guide is published annually for HIV therapy.

Mandell, GL, Douglas, Jr., RG and Bennett, JE: Principles and Practice of Infectious Diseases: Antimicrobial Therapy 1993/1994. Also quite good, and cross-referenced to the definitive textbook in infectious diseases.

Bennett, WM, et al: Drug Prescribing in Renal Failure: Dosing Guidelines for Adults, ed 3. American College of Physicians, Philadelphia, 1994. A concise guide for adjusting medications in renal insufficiency and dialysis.

Medical History and Thought

Ackerknecht, EH: A Short History of Medicine. Johns Hopkins, Baltimore, 1982. The best concise history; enjoyable reading that puts what we do into perspective.

Bordley, III, J and McGehee Harvey, A: Two Centuries of American Medicine 1776–1976. WB Saunders, Philadelphia, 1976. An excellent history.

King, LS: Medical Thinking: A Historical Preface. Princeton University Press, Princeton, NJ, 1982. Good historical and philosophical perspective.

Starr, P: The Social Transformation of American Medicine. Basic Books, New York, 1982. A history of

American medicine from a sociologic perspective; analytic and provocative.

Feinstein, AR: Clinical Judgment. Williams & Wilkins, Baltimore, 1967. The first and most important attempt to evaluate medical thinking in quantitative terms, with good historical analysis.

Rosenberg, CE: Explaining Epidemics: And Other Studies in the History of Medicine. Cambridge University Press, Cambridge, 1992. A collection of thoughtful essays relating to medical history, institutions, and thinking.

Berger, J and Mohr, J: A Fortunate Man. Pantheon, New York, 1967. An essay and photo-essay describing the days of a remarkable English primary-care physician. Good for when you've got the blues or when you're wondering why we're doing all this.

Broyard, A: Intoxicated by My Illness: And Other Writings on Life and Death. Clarkson Potter, New York, 1992. The subjective experience of a terminal illness, as described by a former book reviewer at *The New York Times*.

Osler, W: The hospital as a college. In Aequanimitas: With Other Addresses to Medical Students, Nurses and Practitioners of Medicine. Blakiston, Philadelphia, 1904. The master lays out the reasons and wherefores for teaching medical students in the hospital.

ENVOI

"A contracted view of Medicine naturally confines a man to a very narrow circle, and limits him to a few partial indications in the cure of disease. He soon gets through his little stack of knowledge; he repeats over and over again his round of prescriptions, the same almost in every case; and, although he is continually embarrassed, has the vanity to believe that, from the few maxims which he has adopted, he has within himself all the principles of medical knowledge, and that he has exhausted all the resources of art. This is a notion subversive of all improvement. It flatters the imagination of the indolent, as it dispenses with those toilsome labours which are necessary to the production of truth; and chains him down to a dangerous routine of practice, unworthy the name of art."

—J Morgan, A Discourse Upon the Institution of Medical Schools in America (1765)

Index

Numbers followed by an "f" indicate figures; numbers followed by a "t" indicate tabular material.

A B C Van Dimals (mnemonic), 88–89
Abbreviation(s)
  for diagnoses, 365t
  general principles of, 360
  for medications, 78–79, 366t
  in orders, 360–361t
  for physical findings, 362t
  in prescriptions, 360–361t
  for procedures and operations, 364–365t
  in radiology, 364t
  for symptoms, 362t
  for tests, 362–363t
Abdominal pain
  acute, 188
  definition of, 194
  differential diagnosis of, 194–196
  life-threatening conditions involving, 197
  lower, with rectal bleeding, 197
  management of, 196
Abscess, cough and, 217
Absolute contraindication(s), 100
Academic environment, creation by resident, 5
Access to care, 125
ACE. *See* Angiotensin converting enzyme
Acne, 225
ACP Journal Club, 139
Activity level
  in admission orders, 90
  deep venous thrombosis and, 91
  orders about, 86
Acute abdominal pain, 189
Acute interstitial nephritis (AIN), 198
Acute pericarditis, 172–173
Acute pyelonephritis, 49–50
Acute renal failure (ARF)
  definition of, 198
  differential diagnosis of, 198–199
  localization of, 200
  management of, 199–200
  postrenal causes of, 198–201
  prerenal causes of, 198–200
  renal causes of, 198–200
Addressing patient, 119
Administration, responsibilities of intern, 4
Admission note(s), 35–43, 52–56
Admission order(s), 88–91
Advance directive(s), 127–128

Advanced life support, 127
AG. *See* Anion gap
Age of patient, dosing medication by, 74
Aide, 9
AIN. *See* Acute interstitial nephritis
Airborne route, of transmission of infectious disease, 108
Alanine aminotransferase. *See* Serum glutamic-pyruvic transaminase
Albumin, blood test for, 160
Alkaline phosphatase, blood test for, 159
Allergy
 to medications, 91
 rash in, 222
Altered mental status
 competence issues with, 126–127
 definition of, 201–202
 differential diagnosis of, 202–203
 in elderly, 205
 management of, 203–205
Aluminum hydroxide, 79
Alveolar edema, 166–167
Alveolar infiltrate, 164
Ambulatory medicine
 clinics, 14–15
 emergency department, 17–18
 general principles of, 11–13
 inpatient medicine vs., 11–13
 neighborhood health centers, 16
 physician offices, 16–17
 telephone calls, 18–20
Ambulatory patient, fever in, 181
Ambulatory setting, 11
American Hospital Formulary Service Drug Information, 87
Aminoglycoside, 74
Aminophylline, 77, 81
Analgesic(s), 187–189
 continuous intravenous infusion of, 188
 contraindications to, 196
Anemia
 definition of, 206
 diagnostic template for, 312–313
 differential diagnosis of, 206–207
 management of, 207–208
Anemia of chronic disease, 209
Angina, 172–173, 189–191
Angiotensin converting enzyme (ACE), 349–354, 349t
Anion gap (AG, "delta"), 157–158
Annual physical, 152
Antibiotic(s), 77, 184
 preoperative, 92
 prophylactic, 92
Anticonvulsant(s), 96
Antidepressant(s), 98
Antiepileptic agent(s), 76
Antipyretic(s), 183
Antiviral agent(s), 74
Apical lordotic chest film, 163
Appendicitis, 197
ARF. *See* Acute renal failure
Arterial blood gas, 84
Arterial puncture, 104–105
Arthralgia, 218
Arthritis, 218
Aseptic meningitis, case study of, 355–359
Aspartate aminotransferase. *See* Serum glutamic-oxaloacetic transaminase
Aspiration diet, 86t
Assessment section
 of admission notes, 40–42, 55–56
 of progress notes, 43–44
Asterixis, 206
Atenolol, 93

Atopic atrial rhythm, 168
Atrial fibrillation, 168–169, 185
Atrial flutter, 169
Attending, 4–5
  in ambulatory setting, 13
  personal, 7
  responsibilities of, 6
  service, 6
  teaching, 6
Attending of record, 7
Attending Rounds, 24–25, 130
Axis, of electrocardiographic waves, 170
AZT, prophylactic, 116

Back pain, case study of, 309–315
Barbiturate(s), 75–76
Bayes' theorem, 260–261
Beeper, 72, 123
Beneficence, 123–124
Benzodiazepine(s), 76
Bias, 146–147
Bicarbonate, blood test for, 157
Biliary colic, 197
Bilirubin
  blood test for, 160
  direct, 160, 289–293
  indirect, 160, 289–293
Biochemistry profile, 156–162
Biphasic P wave, 171
Bladder outlet obstruction, 200
Blister, 224
Blood level, of medications, 76
Blood test(s), 151–152
  interpretation of, 154–162
Blood urea nitrogen (BUN), 158
Blood urea nitrogen to creatinine (BUN/Cr), 158
Blood-borne disease, 109–111
Body secretions, disposal of, 111
Body surface area, dosing medication by, 74
Body weight
  dosing medication by, 74
  record of, 33
Bone(s), in chest x-ray, 163
Boolean algebra, 142
Borderline personality disorder, 120–121
Brain death, 202
Brilliant guess, 241–242
BRS Colleague, 141
Bulla, 221, 223–224
Bullous impetigo, 224
Bullous pemphigoid, 223
BUN. *See* Blood urea nitrogen
Bundle branch block, 171–172

Calcium, blood test for, 161–162
Cancer chemotherapeutic agent(s), 74, 77, 81–82
Capsaicin, 188
Captopril test, 213
Carcinoembryonic antigen (CEA) test, 335–340
Cardiac enzyme(s), 191
Cardiomegaly, 165
Cardiopulmonary resuscitation, 127–128
Cardiovascular pressor(s), 74, 77, 81
Care, in doctor-patient relationship, 118
Case presentation(s), formal, 63–66
Case report, 144
Case series, 143–146
Case-control study, 145
Catheter
  central venous, 82
    placement of, 105
  intravenous, placement of, 104
  for intravenous fluids, 81–82
  peripheral, 81–82

Cavitation, 165
CBC. *See* Complete blood count
CEA test. *See* Carcinoembryonic antigen test
Ceftriaxone, 79
Cellulitis, 224
Central venous catheter, 82
  peripherally inserted, 82
  placement of, 105
    procedure note for, 46–47
Characteristic cluster of findings, 235
"Chart Rounds," 25, 130
Chest pain
  definition of, 189
  differential diagnosis of, 189–190
  life-threatening conditions involving, 191
  management of, 190–191
  quantification of, 31
Chest x-ray
  cardinal findings on, 164–167
  interpretation of, 162–167
  protocol for looking at films, 163–164
  techniques in, 163
Chickenpox, 112, 221, 319
Chief complaint, 36–37, 52
Chloride, blood test for, 157
Cholangitis, 197
Cholecystectomy, outpatient note for, 51–52
Cholecystitis, 197
Cholesterol, blood test for, 162
Chorea, case study of, 323–327
Chronic fatigue syndrome, 210–211
Chronic obstructive pulmonary disease (COPD), 84
Chronic pain, 188
CK. *See* Creatine kinase
Clear liquids, 86t, 93
Clerkship, 7, 62
Clinic, 14–15
Clinical case, 279–359
  approach to studying, 278
Clinical problem(s)
  approaches to, 174–175, 284, 288, 314
  case studies of, 279–359
  inpatient, 175–209, 175t
  outpatient, 175t, 209–227
  ranking of, 238
  types of, 233–235
Clinical problem solving, 231–233
  problem list, 233–239
Clinical significance, 146
Clinical trial, 144–145
Clonidine, 93
Closed-space infection, 184
Cluster recognition, 235, 247–249, 248f
CNS lupus, 355–359
Cohort study, 145
Colon cancer, case study of, 335–340
Coma, 202
Competence (ability to make decisions), 126–127
Complete blood count (CBC), 32, 154–155
Complication(s), of procedures, 101–102, 104–106
Computer
  literature search by, 140–143
    medical subject headings, 141
    subheadings, 142
  on-line ordering, 72
  textbooks on, 138
Concurrent medication(s), 74–75
Condition
  in admission orders, 90
  critical, 90
  explaining to patient, 118
  occult, tests to evaluate, 151
  stable, 90
  suspected, tests to evaluate, 151

Confidentiality, 22, 122–123, 125
Confusion, 202, 206
Congestive heart failure, 166
  diet in, 85t
Consensus recommendation, 139
Consent
  informed. *See* Informed consent
  in life-threatening emergency, 126
  for research, 129
Consultant, 7
Consultation, 137–138
  in ambulatory medicine, 12
Contact dermatitis, 223
Contact route, of transmission of infectious disease, 107
Continuity of care, 15
Contraindication(s), to procedures, 100, 104–106
  absolute, 100
  relative, 100
Controlled substance(s), 20, 95
Coombs' test, 209
COPD. *See* Chronic obstructive pulmonary disease
Coronary artery disease, diet in, 85t
Cost
  of ambulatory medicine, 13
  of tests, 153–154
Cough
  case studies of, 285–288, 341–347, 349–354
  definition of, 215
  differential diagnosis of, 216–217
  management of, 217
Countersignature, on orders, 72–73
CPK. *See* Creatine phosphokinase
Creatine kinase (CK), blood test for, 161, 191
Creatine phosphokinase (CPK), blood test for, 161
Creatinine, blood test for, 158
Creme, 77
Critical condition, 90
Critical reading, 143–150
Cut-off analysis, 263–264
Cyst, 220

D5W. *See* 5% Dextrose in water
Daily medication, 77
Daily order(s), 91–92
Day's schedule
  in medicine, pediatrics, or neurology, 130–131
  in surgery or ob/gyn, 131
Decision analysis, 273–274
Dedication, in doctor-patient relationship, 117
Deep venous thrombosis prophylaxis, 91
Delirium, 202, 206
"Delta." *See* Anion gap
Dementia, 202, 206
Dermatitis
  contact, 223
  herpetiformis, 223
  seborrheic, 224
Descriptive study, 144
5% Dextrose in water, 80
Diabetes
  D5W in, 80
  diet in, 85t
Diagnosis, 253
  abbreviations for, 365t
  abnormal vs. normal variation, 276
  in admission orders, 90
  in ambulatory medicine, 11–12
  coherence of, 271
  completeness of, 271
  decision and, 272–274
  differential. *See* Differential diagnosis

Diagnosis (*continued*)
economy of, 271
general principles of, 267–271
histologic-based, 275
power of naming, 270
prior, 235
probabilistic thinking in, 276
problems in, 274–277
readings and references about, 368–370
role in prognosis, 270
threshold for treatment, 272
unifying, 271
Diagnostic template, 243–246, 243–244f
format of, 246
organized by anatomic classification, 245
organized by pathophysiology, 245
Diagnostic testing, 270–271
choosing tests, 261–262
combining tests, 264
continuous values, 263–264
general principles of, 253–254
test characteristics, 255–257, 257f
using tests, 257–261
Diet, orders for, 85–86, 85–86t, 92–93
Dietician, 9
Differential diagnosis, 270
by brilliant guess, 241–242
by cluster recognition, 247–249, 248f
definition of, 240
by diagnostic template, 243–247, 243–244f
general principles of, 240–241
by mnemonic device, 242–243
readings and references about, 368–370
by simple list, 242
strategies for, 241–252
summary of, 251–252
systems approach to, 249–251
by what crosses the mind, 241
Digoxin, 76, 96
Diltiazem, 93
Diphtheria, 269
Diphtheria, pertussis, polio vaccination, 114
Direct bilirubin, 160, 289–293
Dirty utility room, 111
Discharge note(s), 49–50
Discoid lupus, 225
Disease, 267–268, 275
Dispensary, 14
Disposable attire, 109–110
Disseminated infection, rash in, 225
DNR status, 26–27, 128
Doctor. *See* Physician
Doctor-patient relationship
addressing patient, 119
dedication in, 117
ethical responsibilities in, 122–125
interpersonal relations in, 118–122
legal responsibilities in, 125–129
physician unease in
patient causes of, 120–121
physician causes of, 121–122
principles of, 117
respect in, 117, 119
Documentation, 125–126
responsibilities of intern, 4
Droplet spread, 107
Drug(s). *See* Medication(s)
Drug Enforcement Administration number, 95
Drug Facts and Comparisons, 87

Drug Interactions and Side Effects Index, 88
Drugs of Choice, 87
Dyspnea
- definition of, 191
- differential diagnosis of, 192–193
- life-threatening conditions involving, 194
- management of, 193–194
- subjective, without tachypnea, 194

Eczema, 224
Educated guess, estimating pretest probability from, 254
Effective physician-in-training, 132–134
EKG. *See* Electrocardiogram
Elderly, altered mental status in, 205
Electrocardiogram (EKG)
- axis of waves, 170
- cardinal findings on, 172–173
- heart rate, 167–168, 168t
- heart rhythm, 168–169
- interpretation of, 167–173
- intervals, 169–170
- leads, 173
- P-wave morphology, 170–171
- QRS morphology, 171–172
- readings and references about, 371–372
- ST-segment morphology, 172
- T-wave morphology, 172

Emergency, legal issues in, 126
Emergency department, 17–18
Empiric treatment, 180
Enalapril, 93
Encephalopathy, metabolic, 203, 205–206
Endotracheal tube, 84
Enema, preoperative, 92
English language, patient not fluent in, 128–129
Enteric precautions, 111–112
Eosinophil(s), in urinary sediment, 200–201
Erythema, 221
Erythema infectiosum. *See* Fifth disease
Erythema multiforme, 225–226
Erythrocyte sedimentation rate (ESR), increased, 313
ESR. *See* Erythrocyte sedimentation rate
Ethical responsibility, in doctor-patient relationship, 122–125
Ethnicity, 37
Etiology, assessing literature relating to, 148
Exanthem subitum. *See* Roseola infantum
Expert opinion, 137–138
Expertise of physician, 124
Eyewear, protective, 110

Face mask, 82–83
Facial tent, 84
Fairness, 125
False-negative test, 256–257, 256–257f
False-positive test, 152, 256–257, 256–257f
Family history, 30, 53, 334
Family member, physician caring for relatives, 119–120
Fatigue
- causes of, 211
- definition of, 209
- differential diagnosis of, 210
- management of, 211
- medications that cause, 211

Fellow, 5
Fentanyl, 93

Fentanyl patch, 188
Fever
  in ambulatory patient, 181
  case studies of, 285–288, 317–321, 341–347, 349–354
  causes of, 181–182
  definition of, 178
  differential diagnosis of, 178–179
  empiric treatment of, 180
  extreme temperature elevation, 182
  with HIV infection, 182
  in hospitalized patient
    noninfectious, 181
    sustained, 181
  management of, 179–180, 183–184
  postoperative, 182–183
  with rigors, 182
  Tmax, 183
Fever of unknown origin (FUO), 181–182
Fifth disease, 222
  case study of, 317–321
"First, do no harm," 124
First-degree heart block, 169
Fluid(s), intravenous
  catheters used for, 81–82
  KVO, 81
  orders for, 80–82, 92
  preoperative, 92
  rate of administration of, 80–81
  types of, 80
"Focused," 174
Folliculitis, 225
Food, contaminated, 107
Formal case presentation(s), 63–66
Friend, physician caring for own, 119–120
Full liquids, 93
FUO. *See* Fever of unknown origin
Furosemide, 79
Gallbladder pain, 197
gamma-glutamyltransferase (GGT), 159–160
Gastrointestinal bleeding, case study of, 281–284
General therapy, 268
Generic name, 74, 95–96
Generic substitution, 95–97
GGT. *See* gamma-glutamyltransferase
Globulin, blood test for, 160–161
Gloves, 109–110, 115
  sterile, 110
Glucose, infusion in altered mental status, 204
Glucose-6-phosphate dehydrogenase deficiency, case study of, 299–302
Glutamic-oxaloacetic transaminase. *See* Serum glutamic-oxaloacetic-transaminase
Glutamic-pyruvic transaminase. *See* Serum glutamic-pyruvic transaminase
Gold standard, 255, 346
Gown(s), 110
Graduate staff, 5
Grand Rounds, 27
Granular cast(s), in urinary sediment, 200
Grateful Med, 141
Group practice, 16
Guide to Antimicrobial Therapy, 88

Handwashing, 109
Handwriting, legible, 72
Haptoglobin, 209
Hardware, orders about, 87
HDL. *See* High-density lipoprotein
Health care proxy, 103, 128

Health screening, in ambulatory setting, 13
Health-care worker(s)
  with contagious disease, 108
  preventing injury to self, 112–114
  vaccination of, 114
Heart. *See also* Electrocardiogram
  in chest x-ray, 164
  enlarged chambers, 165–166
Heart block
  first-degree, 169
  second-degree
    type I, 169
    type II, 169
  third-degree, 170
Heart murmur, quantification of, 32
Heart rate, 167–168, 168t, 176–177
Heart rhythm, 168–169
Heat rash. *See* Miliaria
Hematocrit, 155, 206
Hematuria, progress note for, 58–61
Hemoglobin level, 155
Heparin, 76–77, 81, 91
Heparin lock, 81–82
Hepatitis A, 111
Hepatitis B, 113
Hepatitis B vaccination, 114
Hep-lock, 81–82
Herpes simplex rash, 223
Herpes zoster. *See* Shingles
High QRS amplitude, 171
High-density lipoprotein (HDL), 162
Histology, 275
History, 29
  in admission notes, 36
  readings and references about, 373–374
History of present illness (HPI), 37–38, 52–53
HIV
  fever in infected patient, 182
  past medical history, 38
  preventing infection of health-care workers, 114–116
  transmission of, 113, 115
"Hold" order, 78
Honesty, in doctor-patient relationship, 119
Hospital
  admission to, routine tests for, 152
  ambulatory vs. hospital care, 11–13
  clinics in, 14–15
  emergency department of, 17–18
  organization of, 3–10
Hospitalized patient
  fever in, 182
    noninfectious, 181
    sustained, 181
  rash in, 226–227
  renal damage in, 201
House officer(s), 5
HPI. *See* History of present illness
Human immunodeficiency virus. *See* HIV
Hydromorphone, 93
Hydroxyurea, 76
Hypercalcemia, diagnostic template for, 311–312
Hypercholesterolemia, outpatient note for, 51–52
Hypertension
  acute secondary complications of, 214
  chronic secondary complications of, 214
  definition of, 212
  differential diagnosis of, 212
  drug-induced, 215
  duration of, 212–213
  isolated systolic, 215
  management of, 212–215
Hypopigmentation, 221

Hypotension
assessment of severity of, 176
definition of, 175
differential diagnosis of, 175–176
management of, 176–178
orthostatic, 177–178
case study of, 281–284
Hypothesis, 231–232, 237, 240, 276

Idioventricular rhythm, 169
Illness, 268, 275
Impetigo, 224–225
Index Medicus, 140
Indication(s), for procedures, 100, 104–106
Indirect bilirubin, 160, 289–293
Infection
closed-space, 184
involving synthetic materials, 184
nosocomial. *See* Nosocomial infection
Infectious disease
health-care worker with, 108
prevalence of, 108
susceptibility to, 108
transmission of, 107–108
Infectious mononucleosis, 320
Infiltrate, in lung fields, 164
Influenza vaccination, 114
Informed consent, 126
for procedures, 102–103, 102t
Infusion pump, 81–82
Inpatient problem(s), 175–209, 175t
Insect bite, 222
Insulin, 76, 93
Intern, 3–4
notes written by, 29
practicing internship, 8
responsibilities of, 4, 10
Interpersonal relations. *See* Doctor-patient relationship
Interstitial edema, 166
Interstitial infiltrate, 164
Interval(s), electrocardiographic, 169–170
Interventional study, 144–146
Interviewer bias, 147
Intramuscular medication, 77, 93
Intravenous (IV) catheter, placement of, 104
Intravenous (IV) fluid(s). *See* Fluid(s), intravenous
Intravenous (IV) medication, 76, 93
IV infusion, 77
IV push, 76
IV Soluset, 77
Inverted P wave, 171
Iron deficiency anemia, 208–209
Isolated systolic hypertension, 215
Isolation procedure(s), 111–112
Itching, case study of, 295–298
IV. *See* "Intravenous" entries

Jaundice, case studies of, 289–293, 295–302
Joint pain
definition of, 218
differential diagnosis of, 218–219
management of, 219
Journal(s), 138
critical reading of, 143–150
reporting on article you have read, 148–150
types of, 138–140
Journal Watch, 139
J-point elevation, 173
Junctional rhythm, 168

Kerley B line(s), 166
Kidney function. *See* Renal function
Knowledge Finder, 141
Known medical condition, 235
Kuru, 112
KVO (keep vein open), 81

Label, on prescription medication, 96
Laboratory specimen, handling and disposal of, 111
Laboratory test(s). *See* Test(s)
Lactate dehydrogenase (LDH), blood test for, 161, 191
Lactated Ringer's solution, 80
Language
  patient who cannot speak English, 128–129
  in written notes, 31
Lateral chest film, 163
Lateral decubitus chest film, 163
LDH. *See* Lactate dehydrogenase
LDL. *See* Low-density lipoprotein
Lead(s), electrocardiographic, 173
Left atrial enlargement, 165–166
Left bundle branch block, 171
Left ventricular enlargement, 165
Left ventricular hypertrophy, 171
Legal record, 30
Legal responsibility, in doctor-patient relationship, 125–129
Legible handwriting, 72
Lichen planus, 223
Lichen simplex chronicus, 224
Lifestyle modification, 212
Listening to patients, 118
Literature. *See* Medical literature
Literature review journal, 139–140
Liver failure, diet in, 86t
Liver function, dosing medication by, 76
Local anesthetic(s), 188
Localized pain, 186
Low-cholesterol diet, 85t
Low-density lipoprotein (LDL), 162
Low QRS amplitude, 171
Lumbar puncture, 105
  procedure note for, 45–46
Lumping and splitting, 237–238, 284
Lung
  in chest x-ray, 164
  open lung biopsy, 349–354, 349t

Macromanagement, 133
Macule, 220–222
Maculopapular eruption, 221–222
Marital status, 39
Mask(s), 115
  protective, 110, 112
MCV. *See* Mean corpuscular volume
Mean corpuscular volume (MCV), 155
Measles, 221, 319
Measles, mumps, rubella vaccination, 114
Mechanical ventilation, 84, 127
Medex, 33, 73
Mediastinum, in chest x-ray, 164
Medical history. *See* History
The Medical Letter on Drugs and Therapeutics, 139–140
The Medical Letter Handbook of Adverse Drug Interactions, 88

Medical literature
  computer literature search, 140–143
  critical reading of, 143–150
  how to use, 371
  problem of quality of, 143–144
  problem of volume of, 143
  readings and references about, 366–374
  reporting on article you have read, 148–150
  sources of information, 137–140
Medical record, 29, 125–126, 128. *See also* Note(s)
Medical student, 7–8
  in ambulatory setting, 13
  as medical team member, 3
  in neighborhood health center, 16
  notes written by, 29
  in physician offices, 17
  responsibilities of, 10
  signing orders, 72
Medical subject heading(s), 141
Medical team, 3
Medical waste, 110
Medication(s)
  abbreviations for, 78–79, 366t
  administration of, 76–77
    after surgery, 93–94
  in admission orders, 90–91
  allergies to, 91
  blood levels of, 76
  concurrent, 74–75
  contaminated, 108
  contraindications to, 88
  dosage of, 74
  dosing intervals, 78
  duration of administration of, 78
  that cause fatigue, 211
  frequency of dosing with, 77–78
  generic names for, 74, 95–96
  that cause hypertension, 215
  interactions of, 88
  labeling of, 96
  notes about, written, 33–34
  orders for, 73–90
  prescriptions for, writing, 94–98
  PRN, 91
  rash caused by, 321
  readings and references about, 87–88, 372–373
  special instructions for, 78
  tolerance to, 76
  trade names for, 74, 95–96
MEDLINE, 140
Melanoma, 333
Meningitis, case study of, 355–359
Mental status, altered. *See* Altered mental status
Meperidine, 188
Meta-analysis, 139, 148
Metabolic encephalopathy, 203, 205–206
Metoprolol, 79, 93
Micromanagement, 133
Miliaria, 223
Mini-MEDLINE, 140–141
Minor, 103, 126
Mnemonic device, 242–243
Monoamine oxidase inhibitor(s), 75
Monoarthritis, 218
Morbilliform eruption, 222
Morning Rounds, 21–22, 130
  presentations on, 66–69
Morning stiffness, 220
Morphine, 79, 93, 188
Multiple myeloma, case study of, 309–315
Multivariate analysis, 147
Murphy's sign, 196
Mycoplasmal infection, 222
Mycosis fungoides, 225
Myocardial infarction, 172, 189–191
Myocardial ischemia, 172

Naloxone, in altered mental status, 204
Narcotic(s), 92, 98
Nasal cannulae, 83
Nausea, case study of, 289–293
Needlestick injury, 113–114
Negative predictive value, 258
Neighborhood health center, 16
Nerve block, 188
Neuropathic pain, 186
Nifedipine, 93–94
Nitroglycerin, 77, 93
Nitroprusside, 76
"No Refill," 95
Nodule, in lung, 165
Nodule (rash), 220, 223
Non-English speaking patient, 128–129
Nonrebreather mask, 83
Nonsteroidal anti-inflammatory drug(s), 187
Normal saline (NS), 80
½ Normal saline, 80
½ Normal saline plus KCl, 80
Normal sinus rhythm, 168
Nosocomial infection. *See also* Infectious disease
  definition of, 107
  general principles of, 107–108
  preventing injury to self, 112–114
  prevention of
    HIV infection, 114–116
    special isolation, 111–112
    Universal Precautions, 109–111, 115
    by vaccination, 114
Note(s)
  admission, 35–43, 52–56
  discharge, 49–50
  do's and don'ts of, 33–35
  general principles of, 29–35
  legal issues in, 125–126
  operative. *See* Note(s), surgical
  outpatient, 50–52
  procedure, 45–47
  progress, 43–44, 57–61
  surgical, 47–49
  update, 44
  written by intern, 4
NPO after midnight, 86t, 92
NPO order, postoperative, 93
NS. *See* Normal saline
Nurse
  carrying out medical orders, 71–72
  responsibilities of, 8–9
  on Work Rounds, 23
Nurse clinician, 8
Nurse practitioner, 8
Nursing assistant, 9
Nursing home admission, routine tests for, 153
Nutrition, artificial, 127

Obstetric patient, routine tests for, 153
Obtundation, 202
Occam's razor, 271
Occult condition, tests to evaluate, 151
Occupation of patient, 38
Occupational therapist, 9
Ointment, 77
Oligoarthritis, 218, 220
On call, 131–132
Open lung biopsy, 349–354, 349t
Operative note(s). *See* Surgical note(s)
Opioid(s), 76, 93, 187
Oral contraceptive(s), 75
Oral medication, 76
Oral presentation(s). *See* Presentation(s)
Order(s)
  abbreviations in, 360–361t
  about activity level, 86
  admission, 88–91

Order(s) (*continued*)
checking correctness of, 87–88
daily, 91–92
for diet, 85–86, 85–86t
flagging of, 73
for fluids, 80–82
general principles of writing, 71
about hardware, 87
how to write, 72–73
by intern, 4
for medications, 73–90
on-line, 72
for oxygen, 82–84
postoperative, 93–94
preoperative, 92
prescriptions, 94–98
renewal of, 92
by telephone call, 72
for tests, 85, 151, 153–154
for treatments, 85
verbal, 72
Order book, 72
Order sheet, 72
Original research, 138
Orthostatic hypotension, 177–178
case study of, 281–284
Outpatient comprehensive health evaluation, 152
Outpatient note(s), 50–52
Outpatient obstetric patient, routine tests for, 153
Outpatient problem(s), 175t, 209–227
Oxygen
blood levels of, 84
delivery of, 82–84, 83t
orders for, 82–84
rate of flow of, 83, 83t
therapy in dyspnea, 193–194
toxicity of, 84

Pain
abdominal. *See* Abdominal pain
back, 309–315
chest. *See* Chest pain
chronic, 188
definition of, 186
joint. *See* Joint pain
localized, 186
management of, 186–187
neuropathic, 186
persistent, 188
phantom, 186
referred, 186
types of, 186
Pancreatitis, 197
Papule, 220–223
Paracentesis, 106
Past medical history (PMH), 38, 53
Patch (rash), 220, 224
Pathophysiology, 243–245
Patience, in doctor-patient relationship, 119
Patient belief, 235
Patient care responsibilities
of attending, 6
of intern, 4
of resident, 5
Patient opinion, 235
Patient-controlled analgesia, 188
PDR. See *Physician's Desk Reference*
Pediatric admission, routine tests for, 152
Pediatric medication, 73
Peer review, 138
Pemphigus vulgaris, 223
Peptic pain, 197
Perforated viscus, 197
Pericardial effusion, 165
Pericarditis, acute, 173
Peripheral catheter, 81–82
Peripheral edema, quantification of, 32
Peripheral pulse, quantification of, 32
Peripheral smear, 209
Peripherally inserted central catheter (PICC line), 82

Peritonitis, 197
Persistent pain, 188
Persistent vegetative state, 202
Personal attending, 7
Personal experience, estimating pretest probability from, 254
Personality disorder, 120–121
Personality of patient, 120–121
Petechiae, 303–307
PGY-1. *See* Intern
PGY-2. *See* Resident
Phantom pain, 186
Phenothiazine(s), 75
Phlebotomist, 9
Phone call. *See* Telephone call
Phosphorus, blood test for, 162
Physical examination
  in admission notes, 36, 39, 54–55
  annual, 152
  in formal case presentation, 64–65
  notes about, 29
  presentation on Morning Rounds, 68–69
Physical finding(s), abbreviations for, 362t
Physical therapist, 9
Physician. *See also* Doctor-patient relationship
  categories in hospital, 3–8
Physician assistant, 8
Physician extender, 8
Physician office, 16–17
Physician's Desk Reference (PDR), 87
Physician-in-training, effective, 132–134
PICC line. *See* Peripherally inserted central catheter
Pityriasis alba, 224
Pityriasis rosea, 225
Plague, 112
Planning section
  of admission notes, 42–43, 56
  of progress notes, 43–44
Plaque (rash), 220, 224–225
Platelet count, 155–156
Pleural effusion, 165
Pleural mass, 165
PMH. *See* Past medical history
Pneumonia
  admission note for, 52–56
  case study of, 285–288
  formal case presentation of, 63–66
  presentation on Morning Rounds, 67–69
  progress note for, 57–58
Pneumothorax, 165
Polyarthralgia without inflammation, 220
Polyarthritis, 218
  symmetric, 219
Porphyria cutanea tarda, 223–224
Portable chest film, 163
Positive predictive value, 258
Posterior probability. *See* Posttest probability
Posterior-anterior chest film, 163
Postinflammatory hypopigmentation, 221
Postoperative care
  diet, 86t, 93
  orders, 93–94
Postoperative fever, 182–183
Posttest probability, 253–254, 257–258, 261–262, 262f, 332, 346, 353
Potassium, blood test for, 156–157
PPD testing, 114
PR interval, 169
Practice format, 16
Practicing internship, 8
Predictive value of test, 258
Preoperative care
  diet, 86t
  orders, 92
Prescription(s), 94–98
  abbreviations in, 360–361t
  how to write, 96–97, 97f
  refills of, 95, 97
  by telephone call to pharmacy, 20

Prescription form, 94–96, 94f
Presentation(s)
 to covering physician at end of day, 70
 formal case, 63–66
 general principles of, 62
 on Morning Rounds, 66–69
 to new member of medical team, 69–70
Pretest probability, 153, 253–254, 258, 261–262, 262f, 266, 345–346, 353
Prevalence
 diagnosis and, 271
 estimating pretest probability from, 254
 of infectious disease, 108
Prevalence study, 144
Prevalence-modifier, 234
Preventive medicine, 13
 outpatient note about, 50
Primum non nocere, 124
Principles and Practice of Infectious Diseases: Antimicrobial Therapy 1993/1994, 88
Prior diagnosis, 235
Prior medication use, dosing medication by, 74
PRN order, 78, 91, 188
Probabilistic thinking, 276
Problem(s). *See* Clinical problem(s)
Problem list
 functions of, 233
 general principles of, 233–236
 preparation of, 236–239
Procainamide, 76
Procedure(s)
 abbreviations for, 364–365t
 complications of, 101–102, 104–106
 contraindications to, 100, 104–106
 indications for, 100, 104–106
 informed consent for, 102–104, 102t
 learning new, 99–100
 performance of, 99–100
  by intern, 4
 readings and references about, 372
Procedure note(s), 44–47
Prognosis, 270
 assessing literature relating to, 147–148
Progress note(s), 43–44, 57–61
Prophylactic antibiotic(s), 92
Propranolol, 93
Prostate, transurethral resection of, surgical note for, 48–49
Protective attire, 109–110
Protein
 blood test for, 161
 dietary, 86t
Psoas sign, 196
Psoriasis, 224–225
Psychiatric admission, routine tests for, 152
Psychiatric illness, 127
Psychosis, 121, 202
Published study, estimating pretest probability from, 254
Pulmonary embolism, 194
Pulmonary infiltrate, 164
Pulmonary vascular congestion, 166
Pulse oximeter, 84
Pustule, 221, 225
P-wave morphology, 170
Pyelonephritis, acute, discharge note for, 49–50

QRS axis, 170
QRS interval, 170
QRS morphology, 171–172
QT interval, 170
Quinidine, 76

Race, 37
Radiology. *See also* Chest x-ray
  abbreviations in, 364t
Randomized clinical trial, 144–145
Rash
  case study of, 317–321
  definition of, 220
  differential diagnosis of, 221–226
  in hospitalized patient, 227
  management of, 226
RBC count. *See* Red blood cell count
Reading, of medical literature, 143–150
Recall bias, 146–147
Rectal suppository, 77, 93
Red blood cell (RBC) cast(s), in urinary sediment, 200
Red blood cell (RBC) count, 154–155
Reference material, 138
Referral, 124
Referred pain, 186
Refill of prescription, 95, 97
Relations with patients. *See* Doctor-patient relationship
Relative contraindication(s), 100
Renal damage
  drug-induced, 201
  in hospitalized patient, 201
Renal dialysis, 127
Renal function. *See also* Acute renal failure
  approximation of, 75
  diagnostic template for renal insufficiency, 313
  dosing medication by, 75
  inadequate perfusion, 201
Renin test, 213
Research
  involving patient in, 129
  original, 139
Research article, assessing quality of, 144
Residency, 5
Resident, 4–5
  on Morning Rounds, 22
Respect, in doctor-patient relationship, 117, 119
Respiratory insufficiency, evaluation for, 193
Respiratory precautions, 112
Restraint(s), 113
Resuscitation status, 26–27
Reticulocyte count, 209
Reverse isolation, 112
Review article, 139
  assessment of, 148
Review of systems (ROS), 39, 53–54
  in formal case presentation, 64
Rickettsia pox, 320
Right atrial enlargement, 166
Right bundle branch block, 171–172
Right ventricular enlargement, 166
Right ventricular hypertrophy, 171
Rocky Mountain spotted fever, 222, 320
ROS. *See* Review of systems
Rosacea, 225
Roseola infantum, 222, 320
Rounds
  Attending, 24–25, 130
  "Chart," 25, 131
  definition of, 21
  Grand, 27
  Morning, 21–22, 66–69, 130
  responsibilities of resident, 5
  "Roundsmanship," 27–28
  Sign-Out, 25–26, 131
  Work, 23–24, 130–131
"Roundsmanship," 27–28
Routine test(s), 151–153
Rubella, 221, 319
"Ruling in," 264
"Ruling out," 264

Saline lock, 81–82
Sarcoidosis, case study of, 349–354
Scabies, 112, 223
Schedule, day's. *See* Day's schedule
Schizophrenia, 121
Screening test(s), 264–266
Scrub typhus, 320
Seborrheic dermatitis, 224
Secondary syphilis, 225
Second-degree heart block
  type I, 169
  type II, 169
Sedative(s), 98
  preoperative, 92
Selection bias, 146
Self-determination, 124–125
Sensitivity of test, 255, 261
Serum glutamic-oxaloacetic transaminase (SGOT), 159, 191
Serum glutamic-pyruvic transaminase (SGPT), 159
Service(s), hospital, 9–10
Service attending, 6
Sexual history, 39
Sexual orientation, 39
Sexual practices, 39
SGOT. *See* Serum glutamic-oxaloacetic transaminase
SGPT. *See* Serum glutamic-pyruvic transaminase
Sharp instrument(s)
  disposable, 110–111
  injuries from, 114–115
  preventing injury to self, 112
Shingles, 221
Sign(s), 234, 240, 247
Signature, on orders, 72–73
Significance
  clinical, 146
  statistical, 146
Sign-out list, 26
Sign-Out Rounds, 25–26, 131
Simple list, in differential diagnosis, 242
Sinus rhythm, normal, 168
Sinus tachycardia, 184
Skin cancer, case study of, 329–333
Skin precautions, 112
Smallpox, 320
SOAP format, 35–36, 43–44, 50
Social history, 38–39, 53
Social worker, 9, 23
Socialization skills, 121
Sodium
  blood test for, 156
  dietary, 85t
Soft tissue, in chest x-ray, 164
Solo practice, 16
Specific therapy, 268
Specificity of test, 255, 261
Spill(s), 111
Sputum staining, 341–347
ST depression, 172
ST elevation, 172
Stable condition, 90
Standard of care, 129
Staphylococcal rash, 222
STAT order, 78
Statistical significance, 146
Status epilepticus, 206
Sterile gloves, 110
Stratification, 147
Streptococcal rash, 222
ST-segment morphology, 172
Student. *See* Medical student
Study design, 144
Stupor, 202
Subcutaneous medication, 77, 93
Subinternship, 8
Sublingual medication, 77, 93–94
Sundowning, 205
Supraventricular tachycardia, 168, 185
Surgical admission, routine tests for, 152

Surgical assistant, 8
Surgical note(s), 47–49
  brief, 48
  complete, 48
Susceptibility to infectious disease, 108
Suspected condition, tests to evaluate, 151
Swallowing problem, 86t
Sydenham's chorea, case study of, 323–327
Symmetric polyarthritis, 220
Symptom(s), 233–234, 236, 240, 247
  abbreviations for, 362t
  quantification in written notes, 31–32
Syndrome, 267–268
Syphilis, 320
  secondary, 225
Systemic lupus, 222
  case study of, 355–359
Systems approach, to differential diagnosis, 249–251

Tachycardia, 168–169
  definition of, 184
  differential diagnosis of, 184–185
  management of, 185
Tall P wave, 171
Tall, peaked T wave, 172
Teaching attending, 6
Technician, 9
Telangiectasia, 221
Telephone call, 18–20
  assessment of medical complaint in, 19
  evaluation of patient by, 19–20
  orders given by, 72
  outpatient note about, 50
  prescriptions to pharmacy by, 20
  recommending therapy in, 19
  relating test data in, 19–20, 50
Tension pneumothorax, 165
Test(s)
  abbreviations for, 362–363t
    in admission notes, 39–40, 55
  assessing literature relating to, 147
  blood. *See* Blood test(s)
  chest x-rays, 162–167
  choice of, 261–262
  combining, 264
  continuous values, 263–264
  costs of, 153–154
  diagnostic, 253–264
  electrocardiogram. *See* Electrocardiogram
  false negative, 256–257, 256–257f
  false positive, 152, 256–257, 256–257f
  fitting into day's schedule, 131
  in formal case presentation, 66
  gold standard, 255
  handling and disposal of laboratory specimens, 111
  interpretation of, general principles of, 151–154
  orders for, 85
    guidelines for, 153–154
    reasons for, 151
  predictive value of, 258
  presentation on Morning Rounds, 69
  readings and references about, 370
  relating data in telephone call, 19–20, 50
  results in written notes, 32
  routine, 151–153
  screening, 264–266, 339

Test(s) (*continued*)
sensitivity of, 255, 261
2 × 2 table, 255–256, 256f, 260–261, 263
true negative, 256–257, 256–257f
true-negative rate, 255
true positive, 256–257, 256–257f
true-positive rate, 255
in update notes, 44
Tetanus immunization, 113–114
Textbook, 138, 368
on computer, 138
Theophylline, 76
Therapy
assessing literature relating to, 148
diagnosis and, 272–274
general, 268
orders for, 85
specific, 268
threshold for, 272
Thiamine therapy, in altered mental status, 204
Third-degree heart block, 169–170
Thoracentesis, 106
Thoracic cavity, in chest x-ray, 164
Thrombocytopenia, case study of, 303–307
"Throwaway," 139
Tinea, 225
Tinea-versicolor, 224
Tmax, 183
Tolerance to medication, 76
Topical medication, 77, 93
Toxic epidermal necrolysis, 224
Tracheobronchitis, 217
Tracheostomy, 84
Tracheostomy collar, 84
Trade name, 74, 95–96
Transbronchial biopsy, 349–354, 349t
Transfusion, in anemia, 208
Translator, 128–129
Transmission of infectious disease, 107–108
Treatment. *See* Therapy
Triage area, 17
Tricyclic antidepressant(s), 75–76
Triglyceride(s), blood test for, 162
True-negative rate, 255
True-negative test, 256–257, 256–257f
True-positive rate, 255
True-positive test, 256–257, 256–257f
Tuberculosis, 108, 112–114
case study of, 341–347
T-wave inversion, 172
T-wave morphology, 172
2 × 2 table, 255–256, 256f, 260–261, 263, 331, 331f
Typhoid fever, 222, 321

Understanding of patient's life, 118–119
Unifying diagnosis, 271
Universal Precautions, 109–111, 115
Update note(s), 44
Ureteral obstruction, 200
Urethral obstruction, 200
Urgent care center, 17–18
Urinalysis, 201
Urinary sediment, 200
Urticaria, 226
Utility room, dirty, 111

Vaccination, of health-care workers, 114
Varicella. *See* Chickenpox
Vasculitis, 222

Vector route, of transmission of infectious disease, 108
Vehicle route, of transmission of infectious disease, 107–108
Venipuncture, 104
Venous compression boot(s), 91
Ventricular fibrillation, 169, 184
Ventricular tachycardia, 169, 184
Verapamil, 93
Verbal order(s), 72
Vesicle, 221, 223
Violent patient, 113
Viral rash, 221–222
Vital signs
  in admission orders, 90
  record of, 33
Vitiligo, 221
Volume depletion, 80

Warfarin, 75–76, 96
Waste disposal, 110
Water, contaminated, 108
WBC count. *See* White blood cell count
Wenckebach's period, 169
Wheal, 221
Wheezing, 194
White blood cell (WBC) count, 154
Withdrawal, altered mental status in, 205
Work Rounds, 23–24, 130–131
Wound precautions, 112
Written note(s). *See* Note(s)
Written order(s). *See* Order(s)

X-ray, chest. *See* Chest x-ray